# Hypertension in
# the Elderly

D0162245

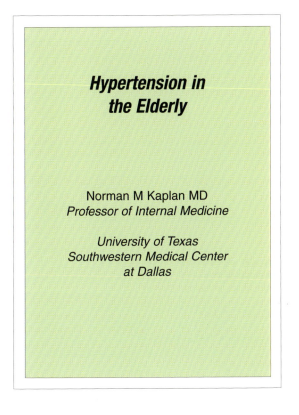

# *Hypertension in the Elderly*

Norman M Kaplan MD
*Professor of Internal Medicine*

*University of Texas
Southwestern Medical Center
at Dallas*

**MARTIN DUNITZ**

The opinions expressed in this book are those of the author and do not necessarily reflect those of Martin Dunitz Limited

© Martin Dunitz Ltd 1999

First published in the United Kingdom
in 1999 by
Martin Dunitz Ltd
The Livery House
7-9 Pratt Street
London NW1 0AE

ISBN 1-85317-729-6

Printed and bound in Spain by Cayfosa

**Contents**

*Introduction* 1

*Mechanisms* 4

*Risks* 16

*Measurement of blood pressure and*
   *postural hypotension* 23

*Evaluation* 37

*The benefits of treating hypertension*
   *in the elderly* 48

*Therapy: lifestyle modifications* 68

*Drug therapy* 78

*Improving compliance* 90

*References* 94

*Index* 101

# Acknowledgements

Figures 19 and 20 are reproduced courtesy of Mr Colin Clements, Kings College Hospital, London.

Figures 21 and 22 are reproduced with kind permission from Beevers DG, MacGregor GA. *Hypertension in Practice*. 2nd Edn. Martin Dunitz, London, 1995

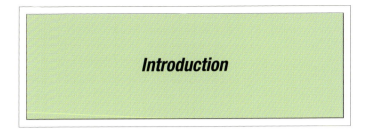

**Introduction**

Before we die, we will probably be hypertensive. With life expectancy now approaching 73 years in men and 80 years in women, the majority of people will develop hypertension before death (Burt et al 1995; Figure1).

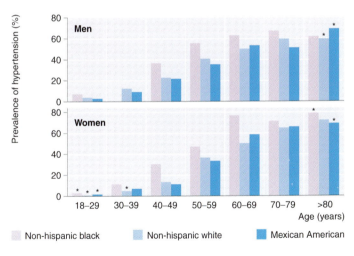

**Figure 1**

*Prevalence of high blood pressure by age and race or ethnicity for men and women in the US population 18 years of age and older. *Estimate based on a sample size that did not meet the minimum requirements of the NHANES III design or relative SEM>30% data from NHANES III. (From Burt et al 1995.)*

Most of this hypertension is pure or isolated systolic hypertension (ISH). In the Framingham Study cohort (Kannel 1998), 60% of those above the age of 65 who had an elevated blood pressure had ISH. This high prevalence of ISH reflects the typical haemodynamic changes occurring with age which raise systolic blood pressure and lower diastolic blood pressure as will be noted later.

The presence of hypertension, be it purely systolic or combined systolic and diastolic, poses a major risk to the elderly, both for mortality, but even more so for morbidity (Kaplan 1998). Hypertension remains the major risk factor for strokes, heart failure, and coronary disease in the elderly, assuming an even greater role than it does in younger people (Table 1).

| Average Annual Rate per 1000 | | | | | | | |
|---|---|---|---|---|---|---|---|
| Ages (years) | All CV events* | | CHD | | Stroke | | CHF | |
| | Men | Women | Men | Women | Men | Women | Men | Women |
| 35–66 | 18 | 9 | 14 | 6 | 3 | 2 | 3 | 2 |
| 65–94 | 43 | 30 | 27 | 17 | 12 | 11 | 11 | 9 |
| Risk ratio (65–94/35–64) | 2.4 | 3.3 | 1.9 | 2.8 | 4.0 | 5.5 | 3.7 | 4.5 |

*Also includes peripheral vascular disease. CV=cardiovascular; CHD=coronary heart disease; CHF=congestive heart failure. (From Kannel 1998.)

**Table 1**
*Increment in risk of cardiovascular events comparing age 35–64 year rates with 65–94 year rates in each sex: 36-year follow-up-Framingham study*

Fortunately, the treatment of hypertension in the elderly will reduce the morbidities associated with the disease, as will be fully described later. Over the relatively short course (3–7 years) of the randomized controlled trials that have documented the value of antihypertensive therapy, the degree of protection against stroke and, even more so, against heart attack has been greater in the elderly than in younger patients. The inherently greater pre-treatment risk status of the elderly provides a greater opportunity for the benefits of blood pressure reduction to be seen than among lower-risk younger patients. Presumably, if younger patients were treated for a much longer period, they would achieve an equal benefit as seen in the elderly over a shorter interval.

Treating the elderly poses a number of special challenges both in diagnosis and in therapy. Fortunately if these challenges are recognized, most can be met and successful therapy can be provided to most elderly hypertensives.

As a clinician who has worked in the field of hypertension for over 30 years, I appreciate the hurdles that practitioners and patients must overcome to manage the disease appropriately. The remainder of this book will provide the details upon which successful management of hypertension in the elderly can be based.

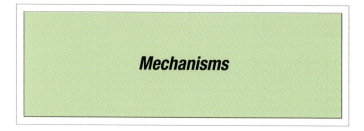

# Mechanisms

Numerous factors, both genetic and acquired, are probably involved in the development of hypertension. Figure 2 (taken from *Clinical Hypertension*; Kaplan 1998) is an attempt to integrate some of these factors into a single scheme of the pathogenesis of hypertension. As research increases our understanding, it has become obvious that no single factor is responsible in the majority of hypertensive subjects. One factor rather than another may be of relatively greater importance in some patients, eg, a reduced nephron number in those who suffered from malnutrition during gestation resulting in intrauterine growth retardation. Factors such as obesity, stress or excess sodium intake may all be of greater importance in some patients.

These various factors are involved in the combined systolic and diastolic hypertension that is typical in middle age and which may carry over into old age. About one-third of hypertension in the elderly is of this type and there is no reason to invoke other pathogenetic mechanisms in those who survive past the age of 65.

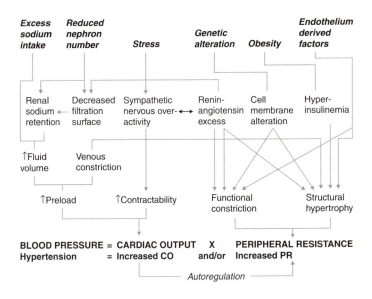

**Figure 2**
*Some of the factors involved in the control of blood pressure that effect the basic equation: blood pressure = cardiac output x peripheral resistance. (From Kaplan 1998.)*

# Renin in the elderly

As we age, a progressive loss of functioning nephrons occurs: only half of the 800 000 nephrons present at birth typically remain at age 70. As the glomeruli sclerose, the juxtaglomerular (J-G) cells lining the afferent arteriole, and which are the source of circulating renin, are also knocked out. In the presence of hypertension an even greater loss of functioning J-G cells accompanies the sclerosis of small arterioles which is the hallmark of hypertensive renal damage: benign nephrosclerosis.

The combination of natural ageing and hypertensive nephrosclerosis reduces the amount of renin secreted from the kidney. Therefore, the circulating renin level measured as plasma renin activity (PRA) typically goes down in the elderly hypertensive. Black patients with hypertension have even lower PRA levels than non-black patients, either because they are born with fewer nephrons or because they are more susceptible to hypertensive nephrosclerosis.

One possible explanation for the greater extent of renal damage in black patients with hypertension is an impairment of kidney development during the latter stages of pregnancy. As proposed by Barker and co-workers (Barker 1995), such intrauterine growth retardation leads to babies who are small for their gestational age. Such small babies grow into adults who have more hypertension, diabetes and coronary disease.

Brenner and co-workers (Brenner and Chertow 1994) believe that reduced renal development is responsible for the subsequent propensity to hypertension (Figure 3). With fewer nephrons, the reduced filtration surface area (FSA) leads to sodium retention and thereby to a rise in systemic blood pressure and subsequently glomerular hypertension. High intra-glomerular pressure leads to progressive glomerular sclerosis, setting up a vicious circle: more hypertension causes more glomerular sclerosis which causes more hypertension.

This scenario almost certainly plays a role in the increased prevalence of subsequent adult hypertension in babies who are small at birth. Whether it is involved in other patients is uncertain but a tendency for increased renal retention of sodium is likely to be a factor in most hypertension, regardless of how the retention arises.

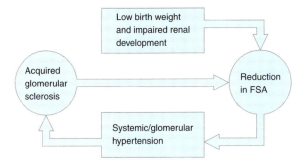

**Figure 3**
*A diagram of the hypothesis that the risks of developing essential hypertension and progressive renal injury in adult life are increased as a result of congenital oligonephropathy, or an inborn deficit of FSA, caused by impaired renal development. Low birth weight, caused by intrauterine growth retardation and/or prematurity, contributes to the oligonephropathy. Systemic and glomerular hypertension in later life results in progressive glomerular sclerosis, further reducing FSA and perpetuating a vicious circle that leads, in the extreme, to end-stage renal failure. (From Brenner and Chertow 1994.)*

The low renin levels of older hypertensives might also reflect their tendency to retain sodium with the subsequent volume expansion raising blood pressure and suppressing the release of renin from the J-G cells.

Regardless of how lower renin levels develop, they probably help to explain why the elderly are more responsive to certain drugs (diuretics and calcium antagonists) and less responsive to other drugs (beta-blockers and angiotensin converting enzyme inhibitors or ACEIs). Their increased response to diuretics probably reflects their greater initial intravascular volume and their slower and smaller rise in renin when the diuretic contracts intravascular volume and lowers blood pressure, two manoeuvres which normally raise renin levels and blunt the continued effect of the diuretic. Since these counter-regulatory forces are less in the elderly, they tend to respond more to the diuretic.

A similar mechanism may be at play with calcium antagonists, whose initial effects include a natriuresis. However, the increased sodium excretion is only transitory and elderly patients may only seem to be more responsive to calcium antagonists because they usually start with higher blood pressure levels which tend to fall more with any antihypertensive therapy.

The smaller response of the elderly to beta-blockers, ACEIs and angiotensin II-receptor blockers (ARBs) probably reflects the fact that all of these agents lower blood pressure at least in part by lowering renin levels or inhibiting renin–angiotensin actions. Therefore, those who start with low renin levels would be expected to respond less to these drugs.

## *Sodium sensitivity*

With fewer functioning nephrons, the elderly hypertensive would be expected to be more sodium sensitive, ie, have a greater rise in blood pressure when given increased dietary sodium and a greater fall in blood pressure when put on a low sodium diet or given a diuretic. Such increased sodium sensitivity has been documented by Weinberger and Fineberg (1991) in a large number of both normotensives and hypertensives put through a rapid test of sodium loading and sodium depletion (Figure 4). With increasing age, both normotensives and hypertensives displayed increasing sodium sensitivity, measured as a greater fall in blood pressure in response to sodium depletion, with the older hypertensives being the most sodium sensitive.

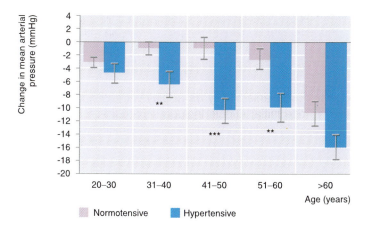

**Figure 4**
*Bar graph showing changes in mean arterial pressure in response to manoeuvres used to define salt responsivity as a function of age in normotensive and hypertensive patients. Standard deviation of the mean given. Significance values between hypertensive and normal subjects: \*\*P<0.01, \*\*\*P<0.001. (From Weinberger and Fineberg 1991.)*

These data are in keeping with the greater response to a sodium restricted diet in the elderly as will be described later. They certainly point to the usual high sodium intake that most people in modern industrialized societies ingest as a contribution to the development of the hypertension that steadily increases among them.

## Systolic hypertension

A different scenario probably explains the progressive rise in systolic blood pressure that is the usual form of hypertension in the elderly (Figure 5). Systolic blood pressure progressively rises after the age of 50 whereas diastolic blood pressure tends to fall. Part of the fall in the average diastolic blood pressure of the population past the age of 50 can be attributed to the early death from cardiovascular disease of those with significantly high diastolic blood pressure. The remainder of these diastolic falls with age probably reflects the basic structural change in the large arteries, the capacitance vessels, which occurs in most people living in industrialized societies, ie, progressive atherosclerosis (Figure 6). Because of the reduced calibre of these capacitance vessels, the normal drain-off into the peripheral vasculature during diastole would leave less blood filling those vessels, reducing the pressure within them.

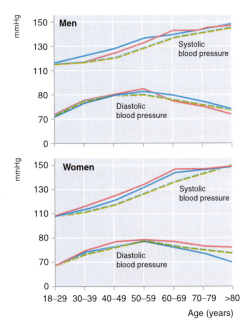

**Figure 5**
*Mean systolic and diastolic blood pressures by age and race or ethnicity for men and women in the US population 18 years of age and older. Data from NHANES III survey. (From Burt et al 1995.)*

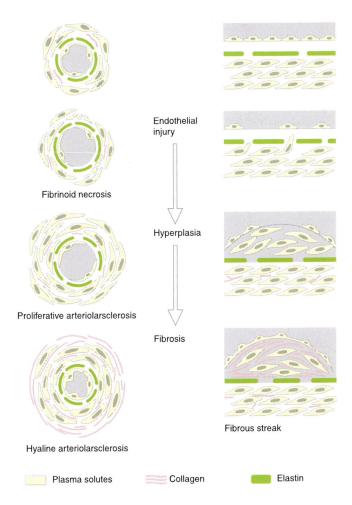

Endothelial
injury

Hyperplasia

Fibrosis

Fibrinoid necrosis

Proliferative arteriolarsclerosis

Hyaline arteriolarsclerosis

Fibrous streak

Plasma solutes    Collagen    Elastin

*Figure 6*
*Small vessel arteriosclerosis, or arteriolar sclerosis (left) has many features in common with large vessel atherosclerosis (right). The diagram outlines mechanisms whereby both lesions might originate from a common source (endothelial injury), which leads to the entry of serum factors that stimulate replication of smooth muscle cell in the intima and formation of an atherosclerotic plaque. In small vessels, the result is hypertrophy, hyperplasia and fibrosis of the vascular media. (From Schwartz and Ross 1984.)*

The basic mechanism for the progressive rise in systolic blood pressure with age is the same loss of distensibility and elasticity in the large capacitance vessels from atherosclerosis. The process was demonstrated over 60 years ago in a simple experiment by Hallock and Benson (1937) (Figure 7). They infused increasing volumes of saline into the tied-off aortas taken from people at autopsy whose ages ranged from the early 20s to the late 70s. The pressure within the aortas from the elderly subjects rose much higher with small increases in volume compared to younger subjects, reflecting the rigidity of the elderly arteries. A volume little more than normal cardiac output was enough to raise pressure significantly, mimicking the situation during life.

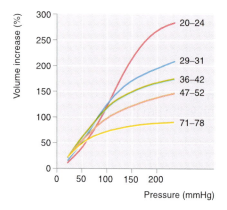

**Figure 7**
*The curves show the relation of the percentage of the increase in volume to the increase in pressure for five different age groups and were constructed from the mean values obtained from a number of aortas excised at autopsy. (From Hallock and Benson 1937.)*

With more sophisticated techniques, the large arteries have been recognized to serve as both conduits and cushions, the first to deliver blood with a minimal fall in pressure to peripheral tissues, the second to smooth out 'the pulsations imposed by the intermittently contracting heart so that blood is directed through these tissues in an almost steady stream' (O'Rourke 1995). With ageing and hypertension, alterations in the cushioning function of the larger arteries occur, changes referred to as 'stiffness' or reduced compliance.

These changes in distensibility and pulse wave velocity that occur with age and that are accentuated by hypertension explain the progressively higher systolic pressures in the elderly. As O'Rourke and co-workers (O'Rourke 1995) have shown, the aortic pulse wave velocity typically doubles by the age of 70 as a manifestation of arterial stiffness from the loss of elastic tissue in the vessel wall. As these pulse waves travel more rapidly and are reflected backwards from the periphery, secondary waves are seen during systole in the elderly (Figure 8). The early return of wave-reflection provides a boost to pressure in late asystole, leading to the progressive rise in systolic pressure but a fall in diastolic pressure, widening the pulse pressure. Thereby, typically the blood pressure goes from 120/80 to 170/60 mmHg and often much higher.

## *Endothelial dysfunction*

Over the past 10 years, a virtual explosion of research has transformed our understanding of the vascular endothelium as a passive lining of the blood vessel walls to an active organ, virtually a factory producing various relaxing and constricting factors. The most exciting of the relaxing factors is nitric oxide, whereas endothelin appears to be the major constricting factor. These various factors are normally in equilibrium but imbalances may explain both hypo- and hypertension.

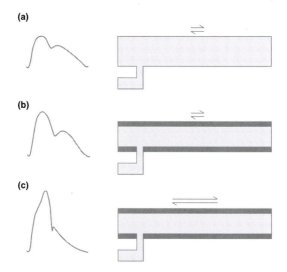

**Figure 8**
*Simple tubular models of the systemic arterial system. (a) Normal distensibility and normal wave velocity; (b) decreased distensibility but normal pulse wave velocity; (c) decreased distensibility with increased pulse wave velocity. At the left are the amplitude and contour of pressure waves that would be generated at the origin of these models by the same ventricular ejection (flow) waves. Decreased distensibility per se increases pressure wave amplitude, while increased wave velocity causes the reflected wave to return during ventricular systole. (From O'Rourke 1995.)*

The endothelial function in otherwise healthy but hypertensive elderly subjects has generally been found to be no different than seen in normotensive elderly subjects. However, endothelial dysfunction as manifested by decreased nitric oxide mediated vasodilatation has been noted in a number of conditions which may afflict the elderly. These include hypercholesterolaemia, glucose intolerance and insulin resistance, and smoking, so it would not be surprising that these contribute to hypertension in the elderly.

## Other mechanisms

Obviously the longer we live, the greater the exposure to various environmental insults which could damage the heart and vasculature and lead to more hypertension. Why only part of the elderly population develop hypertension may reflect differences in genetic endowment or susceptibility to environmental insults. However it arises, hypertension is common and represents the major risk factor for the various cardiovascular complications associated with growing older. The risks imposed by hypertension will be defined next.

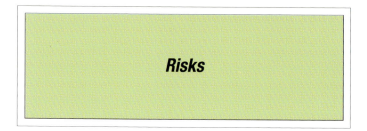

**Risks**

If left untreated, hypertension accelerates atherosclerosis and imposes a further burden on the cardiovascular system (Figure 9). Few of the complications of hypertension seen in Figure 9 are unique to the condition, the obvious exceptions being accelerated-malignant hypertension and hypertensive encephalopathy. These two syndromes were seen in as many as 7% of patients before the advent of effective therapy and were usually fatal. Now they are both less common and much more amenable to effective therapy.

## Age of onset

In most earlier series of patients observed from the presumed onset of primary or essential hypertension, the age of onset was usually before the age of 50. More recently, however, more representative populations have been witnessed wherein as many as 20% of people who developed diastolic hypertension are over the age of 60. As noted earlier, the overwhelming majority of patients who develop isolated systolic hypertension (ISH) are well over the age of 60 and the majority of hypertensives over the age of 65 have ISH.

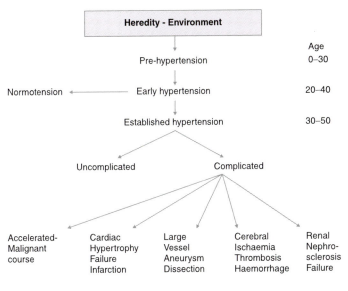

**Figure 9**
*Representation of the natural history of untreated essential hypertension (From Kaplan 1998.)*

In the large population observed by Buck et al (1987) for 5 years after the onset of combined systolic and diastolic hypertension, the rate of the occurrence of cardiovascular events in these newly diagnosed hypertensives was little higher in those in the 40–49 age group as in the 60–65 age group (Table 2). However, the odds ratio of events was far greater in the younger hypertensives than in similarly aged normotensives, whereas the ratio was little different between the older hypertensives and older normotensives: 'Age overtakes hypertension as a cause of cardiovascular disease' (Buck et al 1987).

| Ages group (years) | Rate (per 100)* | | Odds ratio |
| | New hypertensive | Normotensive | |
| --- | --- | --- | --- |
| 40–49 | 4.6 (239) | 0.9 (4677) | 5.2 |
| 50–59 | 5.6 (288) | 3.2 (3655) | 1.8 |
| 60–65 | 6.5 (153) | 5.7 (1301) | 1.2 |

Data from Buck et al 1987
*Number of subjects is shown in parentheses

**Table 2**
*Five-year occurence of cardiovascular events in newly diagnosed hypertensive subjects and normotensive subjects by age at baseline*

## The risks of hypertension in the elderly

None the less, the presence of hypertension poses an additional risk for cardiovascular damage at all ages. Perhaps the clearest portrayal of the progressive increase of both heart attack and stroke with increasing blood pressure is the analysis of MacMahon et al (1990) (Figure 10). Their curves are constructed from data from multiple prospective observational studies in which over 450 000 subjects were followed without therapy for variable periods. These relative risk relationships are for diastolic blood pressure but, as we shall see, the degrees of risk are even steeper for systolic blood pressure.

Note in Figure 10 that the increase in the risk for stroke is steeper than for coronary heart disease (CHD) with every increment in blood pressure but that the number of events, shown as the size of the squares, is much greater for CHD than for stroke. CHD is the leading cause of death in all industrialized societies, but hypertension plays a greater role in the risk for stroke, which is the third leading cause of death overall.

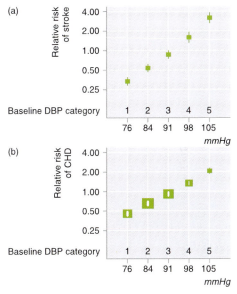

Approximate mean usual DBP (estimated from later remeasurements in the Framingham study)

**Figure 10**

*Relative risk of (a) stroke and (b) CHD, estimated from the combined results of prospective observational studies for five categories of DBP. (Estimates of the usual DBP in each baseline DBP category are from mean DBP values in the Framingham study recorded 4 years after baseline measurement.) The stroke data were obtained from seven prospective observational studies; N=843 events. The CHD data were obtained from nine prospective observational studies; N=4856 events. The solid lines represent disease risk in each category relative to risk in the whole study population (square size is proportional to the number of events in each DBP category). The vertical lines represent 95% confidence intervals for the estimates of relative risk. (From MacMahon et al 1990.)*

Data from one of the studies which provided most of the numbers shown in Figure 11, the Multiple Risk Factor Intervention Trial (MRFIT) in the US, demonstrate the greater relative risk for CHD with increasing systolic blood pressure than for increasing diastolic blood pressure (Neaton and Wentworth 1992). Note the column on the top right representing systolic blood pressure of 160+ and diastolic blood pressure of less than 70 mmHg, the typical pattern of blood pressure in the elderly with isolated systolic hypertension (ISH). This is by far the tallest bar in the figure, documenting the high risk from such elevated systolic levels.

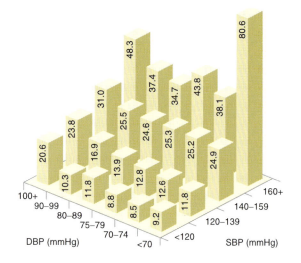

**Figure 11**
*Age-adjusted coronary heart disease death rates per 10 000 person-years by level of SBP and DBP for men screened in the MRFIT.*
*(From Neaton and Wentworth 1992.)*

In multiple placebo-controlled randomized trials involving elderly hypertensives, mortality rates over the 4–5 years of follow-up among those on placebo were similar in those with ISH as in those with combined systolic and diastolic hypertension. Compared to normotensives those with ISH have more coronary disease and even more strokes, with an approximate 1% increase in all-cause mortality rates with each 1 mm rise in systolic pressure.

## *Older versus younger*

The Framingham data (Kannel 1998) show the far greater risk for the elderly than for the younger at all levels of both systolic and diastolic pressure (Figure 12). Women have a lower incidence of cardiovascular disease than men at all ages and with both measures of blood pressure.

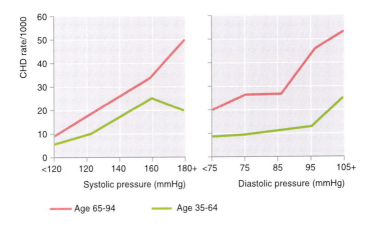

**Figure 12**
*Incidence of coronary heart disease by age and levels of systolic blood pressure for a 30 year follow-up in men in the Framingham study. (From Kannel 1998.)*

# The very old

A possible exception to the progressive risks associated with every rise in systolic pressure has been claimed for the very old, people over the age of 85. Heikinheimo et al (1990) followed 724 non-institutionalized 84–88 year olds in Finland and found the lowest mortality rates were in those with systolic blood pressure of 140–169 mmHg and diastolic pressure of 70–99 mmHg. Others, such as Boshuizen et al (1998), have noted better survival in people aged 85 and older with higher initial systolic and diastolic blood pressure than in those with lower readings. This inverse relation is mainly due to the poor general health that causes low blood pressure in the elderly.

# Hypertension and dementia

Hypertension predisposes the elderly to their major morbidity, dementia. Such dementia is often vascular in origin, reflecting multiple small infarcts throughout the brain. Fortunately, the incidence of dementia has been found to be reduced in elderly hypertensives given antihypertensive therapy. The most striking effect was reported by Forette et al (1998) from the SYST-EUR trial of a long-acting dihydropyridine calcium antagonist, nitrendipine. It is likely that any effective antihypertensive regimen will protect against vascular dementia as it will against strokes, as noted later.

Before considering the ability of antihypertensive therapy to protect the elderly hypertensive, we will consider the measurement of blood pressure and those special features of blood pressure in the elderly, ie, pseudohypertension and postural hypotension.

Of all the routine procedures done in clinical practice, measurement of blood pressure (BP) is surely the one that is least accurate but at the same time most important. According to O'Brien (1996), 'blood pressure measurement as done in clinical practice today is a very inaccurate procedure, yet one on which we base management decisions with serious far-reaching consequences for the patient'.

There is a need for multiple and more accurate blood pressure measurements primarily because of the marked variability of the blood pressure as shown in the 24 h readings taken by an automatic recorder on a single patient taking no medication and performing his usual daily activities (Figure 13). Note the marked difference in the readings taken at 16:30hrs (160/110 mmHg) and the one taken at 13:30hrs (120/62 mmHg). Various extraneous factors could explain this 40/48 mmHg difference between the two readings. These include physical activity, smoking, anxiety, urinary bladder distention, caffeine ingestion and literally a hundred other factors, many of which cannot be controlled and which are usually not considered. Clearly, if only a few (even accurate) values of blood pressure are taken, noticeable over- and underestimates may be obtained. The only way to overcome the problem of variability is to take multiple readings, following the guidelines as carefully as possible (Table 3, Figure 14).

### Patient Conditions

**Posture**
Initially, particularly in patients >65 years, with diabetes, or receiving antihypertensive therapy,
check for postural changes by taking readings after 5 min supine, then immediately upon and 2 min after standing
For routine follow-up, the patients should sit quietly for 5 min with the arm bared and supported at the level of the heart and the back resting against the chair

**Circumstances**
No caffeine or smoking within 30 min preceding the reading
No exogenous adrenergic stimulants (eg, phenylephrine in nasal decongestants)
A quiet, warm setting

### Equipment

**Cuff size**
The bladder should encircle at least 80% of the circumference and cover two-thirds of the length of the arm; if it does not, place the bladder over the brachial artery
A too small bladder may cause falsely high readings

**Manometer**
Either a mercury, recently calibrated aneroid or validated electronic device

**Table 3**
*Guidelines for measurement of blood pressure*

### Stethoscope

The bell of the stethoscope should be used; to avoid interference, the cuff may be placed with the tubing on the top

### Infants

Use ultrasound (eg, the Doppler method)

### *Technique*

### Number of readings

On each occasion, take at least two readings, separated by as much time as is practical; if readings vary by >5 mmHg, take additional readings until two are close

For diagnosis, obtain three sets of readings at least 1 week apart

Initially, take pressure in both arms; if the pressures differ, use the arm with the higher pressure

If the arm pressure is elevated, take the pressure in one leg, particularly in patients <30 years old

### Performance

Inflate the bladder quickly to a pressure 20 mmHg above the systolic pressure, recognized by disappearance of the radial pulse, to avoid an auscultatory gap

Deflate the bladder 3 mmHg/s

Record the Korotkoff phase I (appearance) and phase V (disappearance), except in children, for whom use of phase IV (muffling) may be preferable

If the Korotkoff sounds are weak, have the patient raise the arm and open and close the hand 5–10 times; then inflate the bladder quickly

### Recordings

Note the pressure, patient position, the arm, and cuff size (eg, 140/90 mmHg, seated, right arm, large adult cuff)

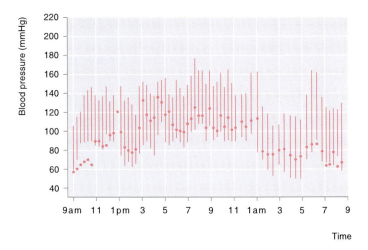

**Figure 13**
*Computer printout of blood pressures obtained by ambulatory blood monitoring over 24 h beginning at 09:00hrs in a 50 year-old man with hypertension receiving no therapy. The patient slept from midnight until 06:00hrs, Heart rate in beats/min. (From Zachariah et al 1988.)*

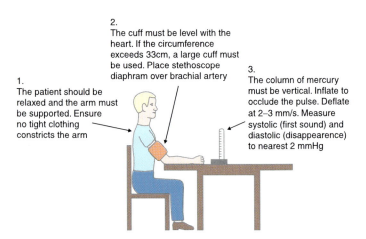

2.
The cuff must be level with the heart. If the circumference exceeds 33cm, a large cuff must be used. Place stethoscope diaphram over brachial artery

3.
The column of mercury must be vertical. Inflate to occlude the pulse. Deflate at 2–3 mm/s. Measure systolic (first sound) and diastolic (disappearance) to nearest 2 mmHg

1.
The patient should be relaxed and the arm must be supported. Ensure no tight clothing constricts the arm

**Figure 14**
*Technique of blood pressure measurement recommended by the British Hypertension Society. (From British Hypertension Society 1985.)*

# The white coat effect

Even if all these guidelines are carefully followed, routine clinical measurements by sphygmomanometry will probably display considerable variability. In particular the 'white coat' effect will often result in higher readings in the office than are obtained outside the office. This 'alerting reaction' is partly in response to the presence of the physician and to a lesser degree to a nurse, but more from the anticipation of going to the doctor's office. A good demonstration of the typical differences between office readings and readings taken by the patient at home with an electronic device is shown in Table 4 (Hall et al 1990). In both the treated and untreated patients, the first set of clinic readings were higher than the second set of clinic readings taken 2 weeks later, showing the usual fall in blood pressure noted on repeated readings over the first few weeks. Even more impressive is the difference between the clinic

| Patient group | First clinic reading (mercury manometer) | | Home series (electronic device) | | Second clinic reading | | | |
|---|---|---|---|---|---|---|---|---|
| | | | | | Electronic device | | Mercury manometer | |
| | SBP | DBP | SBP | DBP | SBP | DBP | SBP | DBP |
| Untreated (n = 114 ) | 174 | 103 | 148 | 90 | 165 | 95 | 164 | 97 |
| Treated (n = 154) | 177 | 104 | 147 | 87 | 163 | 95 | 164 | 95 |
| Data from Hall et al 1990 | | | | | | | | |

**Table 4**
*Blood pressure recorded at home between clinic visits*

readings and the average of 32 self-recorded home readings taken in the 2 weeks between the two office visits, the Home Series in Table 4. The home readings were lower in 80% of the patients, by more than 20/10 mmHg in 40%, so that therapy was deemed unnecessary in 38% of the untreated patients and could be reduced in 16% of the treated ones. The accuracy of the home readings taken with the electronic devices is shown by the identical results with that device and the mercury manometer at the second clinic visit.

## *White coat hypertension*

Although the blood pressure typically falls over the first few weeks of repeated measurements taken either in the office or at home, in about 20–30% of patients the office readings remain elevated but those taken out of the office are normal. This condition is referred to as 'white coat hypertension' or 'isolated clinic hypertension'. This condition was clearly identified by Pickering and co-workers among 292 untreated patients with office readings that were persistently elevated above 140/90 mmHg over an average of 6 years (Pickering 1988). When out-of office recordings were obtained by 24 h ambulatory monitoring, the average daytime reading was below 134/90 mmHg in 21% of the patients.

Similar percentages of white-coat hypertension have been noted in various populations all over the world. Of interest, the prevalence rises with the age of the patient and is particularly high in elderly patients with isolated systolic hypertension. Therefore it is important to obtain out-of-office readings either by self-recorded home measurements or ambulatory automatic monitors if at all possible before diagnosing hypertension in the elderly. Every practitioner should have a few electronic devices to loan to new patients for a few weeks of home recordings. Where feasible, a single 24 h ambulatory recording will suffice, taking the average of all of the daytime readings since those taken during sleep are typically lower (see Figure 13) and should not be used in defining the presence of hypertension.

A number of caveats are to be noted concerning white-coat hypertension.

- The prevalence depends on the definition of the upper limit of normal for daytime out-of-office readings. Mancia et al (1997) recommend 130/85 mmHg, the 95th percentile of a large sample of the population of Monza, Italy.

- A considerable portion of patients considered to be resistant to therapy on the basis of office readings above 140/90 mmHg while on multiple medications have been found to have normal readings when blood pressures are taken out of the office. The appropriate evaluation of such patients is demonstrated in Figure 15. If significant target organ damage is present, more aggressive treatment is indicated even if a white-coat component is making the office pressure higher than it is out of the office. If target organ damage is not present, home blood pressures should be obtained and, if they are low, ambulatory monitoring might be considered to document the 'pseudo-resistance'. Obviously, if home or ambulatory blood pressures are high, true resistance is confirmed and more aggressive therapy should be provided.

- The natural history of white-coat hypertension is under intense scrutiny but has not yet been completely elucidated. Most investigators find a few less than normal features among white-coat hypertensives. However the longest follow-up of a sizeable group of carefully defined patients with ambulatory readings below 130/80 mmHg shows no increase in cardiovascular events among them compared to a group of patients with normal office and ambulatory readings (Verdecchia et al 1996)) (Figure 16).

Note that when Verdecchia et al used a less restrictive higher upper limit of normal to define white-coat hypertension (Group C), many of these patients did suffer a cardiovascular event, their probability being similar to that seen in the patients with ambulatory hypertension (Group D). Clearly, the diagnosis of white-coat hypertension should be restricted to those with truly normal out-of-office readings.

- In keeping with the above caution, if home readings are used, the patient should be instructed to take multiple readings while stressed as well as while relaxed, at home and at work, so as to recognize the true status of the blood pressure. If only relaxed blood pressures are used, many more patients will be thought to have white-coat hypertension than actually do.

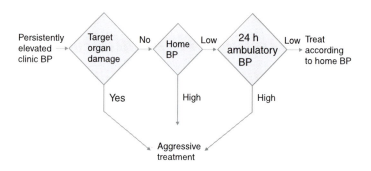

**Figure 15**
*Proposed schema of blood pressure measurement for patients with apparently resistant hypertension. (From Pickering 1988.)*

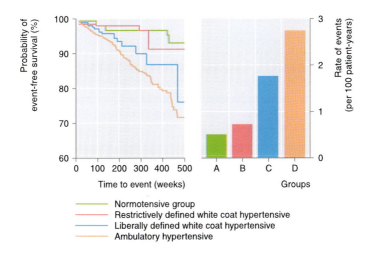

**Figure 16**

*Rate of major cardiovascular morbid events in the normotensive group and in the groups with white coat and ambulatory hypertension. Event rate did not differ between the normotensive group (A) and the group with more restrictivity defined white coat hypertension (B): daytime ambulatory BP<130/80 mmHg. Event rate increased in the group with the more liberally defined white coat hypertension (C). The event rate in group C did not differ from that in the group of patients  with ambulatory hypertension (D). (From Verdecchia et al 1996.)*

As of now, the best course is to obtain out-of-office readings to identify white coat hypertension since those patients cannot be otherwise recognized. If the patient is truly normotensive out of the office, neither should the diagnosis of hypertension be affixed to the patient nor should antihypertensive drug therapy be started.  Rather, such patients should be strongly encouraged to modify harmful lifestyle habits (as will be described later) and to monitor carefully their blood pressure since some may progress to persistent hypertension.

Some investigators and practitioners object to this more conservative approach, noting that all of the data on the risks of hypertension have been based on office readings, and often on only a limited number of them. More long-term follow-up is needed but, at present, out-of-office readings do seem to be more closely predictive of future risk. High office readings are not to be disregarded but they include some with truly high readings (who are at increased risk) and others with readings that are high because of the white-coat effect (who seem to be at little increased risk). Since not all with high office readings suffer subsequent cardiovascular disease, it is very likely that differences in risk reflect the inclusion of both persistently hypertensive and only office elevated readings.

## *Pseudohypertension*

As noted, the white-coat effect is more common and significant in the elderly than in younger people  so out-of-office readings should be obtained, if possible. In addition to white-coat hypertension, the elderly may have artifactually elevated pressures by usual indirect cuff measurements because of increased stiffness of the large arteries, which precludes compression and collapse of the brachial artery. Therefore, the manometer shows much higher pressures in the balloon than are present within the artery, giving rise to pseudohypertension.  The prevalence varies in various reports but is probably less than 5%.  It should be suspected if high sphygmomanometer readings are noted but few signs of such severe hypertension are present and particularly if symptoms of hypotension follow  only modest lowering of pressure by antihypertensive therapy.  More accurate estimates of true intra-arterial pressure may be obtained by automatic infrasonic measurements or finger recordings.

# Posteral and postprandial hypotension

## Definition and incidence

A fall in systolic pressure of 20 mmHg after 1 min of quiet standing is usually taken as an abnormal response indicative of postural hypotension. In the generally healthy population of elderly men and women enrolled in the Systolic Hypertension in the Elderly Program, postural hypotension was found in 10.4% at 1 min after rising from a seated position and in 12.0% at 3 min, with 17.3% having hypotension at one or both intervals. The prevalence would probably have been higher if the patients had been tested after rising from a supine position. The only predisposing factor for postural hypotension found in an unselected elderly population was hypertension. As seen in Figure 17 the higher the basal supine systolic blood pressure, the greater the postural fall.

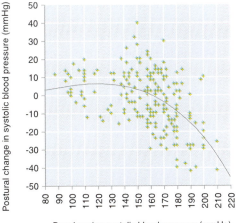

**Figure 17**
*Relationship between basal supine systolic BP and postural change in systolic BP for aggregate data from older subjects. (From Lipsitz et al 1985.)*

## Mechanism

Normal ageing is associated with various changes that may lead to postural hypotension. The two most common in patients with supine or seated hypertension are venous pooling in the legs and autonomic insufficiency. The reductions in baroreceptor sensitivity that often accompany isolated systolic hypertension are mainly related to ageing.

Postprandial hypotension is related to splanchnic pooling of blood after eating. As reported by Grodzicki et al (1998) among 530 patients aged 60–100 years, ambulatory blood pressure monitoring revealed some decreases in both systolic and diastolic pressure in 70%, reaching -16/-12 or more in 24%.

## Management

Postural hypotension must often be treated before the frequently coexisting seated and supine hypertension can be managed. A succinct summary by Tonkin (1995) of the exacerbating factors, pathophysiology and therapy of postural hypotension is shown in Figure 18. A few additional points deserve emphasis.

- A trial of withdrawal of antihypertensive therapy may be worthwhile if simple measures are not effective; however, postural hypotension may improve after effective antihypertensive therapy.

- Simple physical countermeasures often do work, including sleeping with the head tilted up and any isometric exercise but particularly leg crossing and thigh contraction.

- Drugs that may work include the partial $\beta$ agonist pindolol; erthyropoietin; the somatostatin analog octreotide, particularly to prevent splanchnic pooling after eating; and the $\alpha$ agonist midodrine, for those with neurogenic causes.

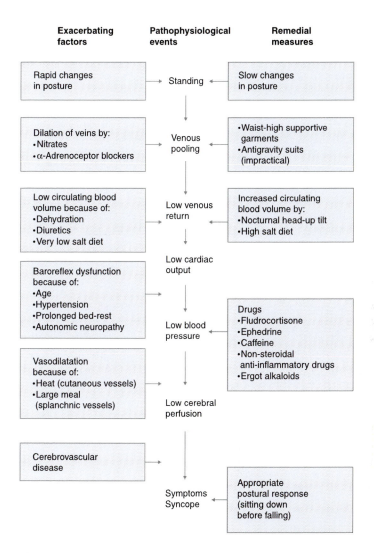

| Exacerbating factors | Pathophysiological events | Remedial measures |
|---|---|---|

**Exacerbating factors** — **Pathophysiological events** — **Remedial measures**

Rapid changes in posture → Standing ← Slow changes in posture

↓

Dilation of veins by:
• Nitrates
• α-Adrenoceptor blockers
→ Venous pooling ← • Waist-high supportive garments
• Antigravity suits (impractical)

↓

Low circulating blood volume because of:
• Dehydration
• Diuretics
• Very low salt diet
→ Low venous return ← Increased circulating blood volume by:
• Nocturnal head-up tilt
• High salt diet

↓

Low cardiac output

↓

Baroreflex dysfunction because of:
• Age
• Hypertension
• Prolonged bed-rest
• Autonomic neuropathy
→ Low blood pressure ← Drugs
• Fludrocortisone
• Ephedrine
• Caffeine
• Non-steroidal anti-inflammatory drugs
• Ergot alkaloids

Vasodilatation because of:
• Heat (cutaneous vessels)
• Large meal (splanchnic vessels)
→

↓

Low cerebral perfusion

↓

Cerebrovascular disease →

↓

Symptoms Syncope ← Appropriate postural response (sitting down before falling)

*Figure 18*

*Summary of the pathophysiological events that occur during the development of symptoms of postural hypertension (middle column) and the interaction of exacerbating factors (left column) and remedial measures (right column) with these events. (From Tonkin 1995.)*

Postprandial hypotension is usually ameliorated by smaller meals, perhaps lower in carbohydrate to minimize the rise in insulin which may induce vasodilation. Caffeine does not prevent postprandial hypotension.

## Definition of hypertension

Now that we have reviewed the proper measurement of blood pressure in the elderly, which obviously must include supine and standing readings, attention will be directed to the remainder of the evaluation in those found to be hypertensive, defined as a usual blood pressure above 140/90 mmHg (Table 5). Those with systolic pressure above 140 and diastolic pressure below 90 mmHg are defined as isolated systolic hypertension (ISH), although in many series ISH is reserved for those with systolic pressure above 160 mmHg.

| Category | Systolic (mmHg) | Diastolic (mmHg) |
|---|---|---|
| Normal† | <130 | <85 |
| High normal | 130–139 | 85–89 |
| Hypertension‡ | | |
|     Stage 1 | 140–159 | 90–99 |
|     Stage 2 | 160–179 | 100–109 |
|     Stage 3 | >180 | >110 |

Data from Joint National Committee 1997.
* These definitions apply to adults who are not taking antihypertensive drugs and who are not actually ill. When systolic and diastolic BP fall into different categories, the higher category should be selected to classify the individual's BP status. Isolated systolic hypertension is defined as SBP > 140 mmHg and DBP<90 mmHg and stage appropriately.
†Optimal BP with respect to cardiovascular risk is <120 mmHg systolic and <80 mmHg diastolic.
‡Based on the average of two or more readings taken at each of two or more visits after an initial screening.

**Table 5**
*Classification of blood pressure for adults aged 18 years and older\**

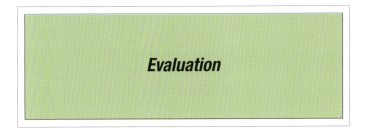

*Evaluation*

There are three main reasons to evaluate patients with hypertension (Kaplan 1998):

1   To determine the type of hypertension, specifically looking for reversible causes

2   To assess the impact of the hypertension on target organs

3   To estimate the patient's overall risk profile for the development of premature cardiovascular disease.

Such evaluation can be accomplished with relative ease and should be part of the initial examination of every newly discovered hypertensive. The younger the patient and the higher the blood pressure, the more aggressive the search for reversible causes should be. Among middle-aged and older patients, greater attention should be directed to the overall cardiovascular risk profile, since these populations are more susceptible to immediate catastrophes unless preventive measures are taken.

# *History*

The patient's history should focus on the duration of the blood pressure and any prior treatment, the current use of various drugs that may cause it to rise and the symptoms

| | |
|---|---|
| **Duration of hypertension** | **Presence of other risk factors** |
| Last known normal blood pressure | Smoking |
| Course of the blood pressure | Diabetes |
| **Prior treatment of the hypertension** | Dyslipidaemia |
| Drugs: types, doses, side effects | Physical inactivity |
| **Intake of agents that may cause hypertension** | **Dietary history** |
| | Sodium |
| Oral contraceptives | Alcohol |
| Sympathomimetics | Saturated fats |
| Adrenal steroids | **Psychosocial factors** |
| Excessive sodium intake | Family structure |
| **Family history** | Work status |
| Hypertension | Educational level |
| Premature cardiovascular disease or death | **Sexual function** |
| | **Features of sleep apnoea** |
| Familial diseases: pheochromocytoma, renal disease, diabetes, gout | Early morning headaches |
| | Daytime somnolence |
| | Loud snoring |
| **Symptoms of secondary causes** | Erratic sleep |
| Muscle weakness | |
| Spells of tachycardia, sweating, tremor | |
| Thinning of the skin | |
| Flank pain | |
| **Symptoms of target organ damage** | |
| Headaches | |
| Transient weakness or blindness | |
| Loss of visual acuity | |
| Chest pain | |
| Dyspnoea | |
| Claudication | |

*Table 6*
*Important aspects of the history*

of target organ dysfunction (Table 6). Though not usually considered part of the initial workup, attention should also be directed toward the patient's psychosocial status, looking for such information as the degree of knowledge about hypertension, the willingness to make necessary changes in lifestyle and to take medication, and the family and job situations. An area of great importance is sexual dysfunction, often neglected until it arises after antihypertensive therapy is given. Impotence, often attributed to antihypertensive drugs, may be present in as many as half of untreated, elderly hypertensive men and is most likely related to their underlying vascular disease.

## *Physical examination*

The physical examination should include a careful search for damage to target organs and for features of various reversible causes (Table 7).

---

Accurate measurement of blood pressure

General appearance: distribution of body fat, skin lesions, muscle strength, alertness

Funduscopy

Neck: palpation and auscultation of carotids, thyroid

Heart: size, rhythm, sounds

Lungs: rhonchi, rales

Abdomen: renal masses, bruits over aorta or renal arteries, femoral pulses

Extremities: peripheral pulses, oedema

Neurological assessment

---

**Table 7**
*Important aspects of the physical examination*

## Funduscopic

Only in the optic fundi can small blood vessels be seen with ease, but this requires dilation of the pupil, a procedure that should be more commonly practised. With the short-acting mydriatic tropicamide 1%, excellent dilation can be achieved in almost 90% of patients within 15 min.

Keith, Wagener and Barker in 1939 originally classified the funduscopic changes but mixed two separate vascular changes: hypertensive neuroretinopathy (hemorrhages, exudates and papilloedema) and arteriosclerotic retinopathy (arteriolar narrowing, arteriovenous nicking and silver wiring). Dodson et al (1996) proposed a simpler grading system for hypertensive retinopathy: A (non-malignant), generalized arteriolar narrowing and focal constriction; and B (malignant), haemorrhages, hard exudates, and cotton wool spots, with or without optic disc swelling (Figures 19 and 20).

# *Laboratory data*

### Routine

As described in the 6th Joint National Committee (1997) report (JNC-6), for most patients, a haematocrit, a urine analysis, an automated blood chemistry (glucose, creatinine, electrolytes), a lipid profile (total and high density lipoprotein cholesterol, triglycerides) and an ECG are all of the routine procedures needed. None of these usually yields abnormal results in the early, uncomplicated phases of essential hypertension; but they should always be obtained for a baseline. Surprisingly, only 17% of general practitioners in several countries routinely obtain even this minimal assessment.

Hypertriglyceridaemia and, even more threatening, hypercholesterolaemia are found more frequently in untreated hypertensives than in normotensives. The prevalence increases with the blood pressure level. The association may, in turn, reflect the quartet of upper body obesity, hyperlipidaemia, glucose intolerance, and hypertension related to hyperinsulinaemia. Lipoprotein (a) levels and certain apolipoprotein (a) isoforms are strong and independent risk factors for coronary disease in hypertensives, so these measurements may be added to the lipid profile.

Hyperuricaemia is found in up to half of untreated hypertensives and reflects underlying nephrosclerosis. Not only is gout more common in hypertensives but so are kidney stones, which are probably a consequence of increased urinary calcium excretion. Incipient renal disease may be heralded by microalbuminuria.

## Testing for target organ damage

Left ventricular hypertension hypertrophy (LVH), if significant in degree, can be identified by ECG (Figure 21). Lesser degrees of LVH are identified by echocardiography but, until the recognition of LVH is shown to add independent prognostic information, echocardiography is not recommended as a routine procedure in view of its cost.

In the presence of symptoms of cerebral ischaemia, the finding of a carotid bruit indicates the need for carotid ultrasonography in the hope of finding a significant and correctable lesion.

Renal dysfunction is usually first recognized by microalbuminuria and testing for this may become routine. Usually, additional testing for renal damage is reserved for those with elevated serum creatinine levels.

Aortic abdominal aneurysms should be looked for by careful palpation and if suspected confirmed by ultrasonography followed by appropriate imaging procedures (Figure 22).

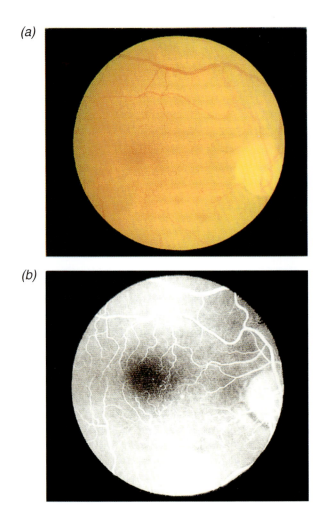

**Figure 19**

*(a) Right eye showing tortuous vessels supero-temporal to the optic disc and some microaneuysms close to the fovea, possibly a microvascular occlusion secondary to hypertension. (b) Fluorescein angiogram in the arteriovenous phase of the same patient, showing the tortuous vessels, microaneurysms and dilated capillaries on the nasal side of the foveal arcade. There is also some capillary 'drop out' indicating early ischaemia.*

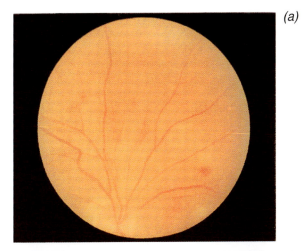

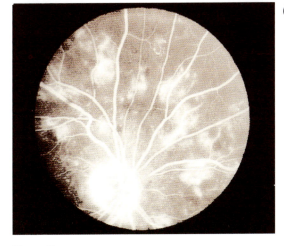

**Figure 20**

*(a) Left eye of patient showing numerous cotton wool spots and haemorrhages supero-nasal to the disc. (b) Fluorescein angiogram in the arteriovenous phase showing masking from the haemorrhages and cotton wool spots. There is leakage from and staining of vessels as they cross poorly perfused areas of the retina. A few microaneurysms can be seen at the top of the picture.*

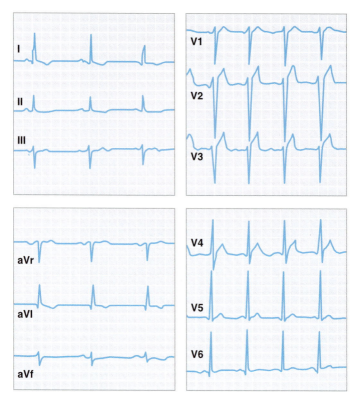

**Figure 21**
*ECG of a patient with left ventricular hypertrophy.*

# Searching for identifiable causes

Evaluation for the major identifiable (or secondary) causes of hypertension is outlined in Table 8. Usually the initial workup for these often reversible causes is limited to patients with features of "inappropriate" hypertension

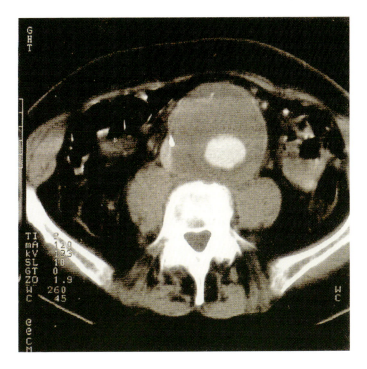

**Figure 22**
*CT scan showing abdominal aortic aneurysm.*

(Table 9). The one most likely to be found in the elderly is atherosclerotic renovascular disease, particularly when hypertension appears or worsens suddenly and develops on the background of extensive atherosclerotic disease

| | Diagnostic procedure | |
|---|---|---|
| **Diagnosis** | **Initial** | **Additional** |
| Chronic renal disease | Urinalysis, serum creatinine, renal sonography | Isotopic renogram, Renal biopsy |
| Renovascular disease | Captopril-enhanced isotopic renogram, duplex sonography | Aortogram |
| Coarctation | Blood pressure in legs | Aortogram |
| Primary aldosteronism | Plasma and urinary potassium, plasma renin and aldosterone (ratio) | Plasma or urinary aldosterone after saline load Adrenal CT and scintiscans |
| Cushing's syndrome | Morning plasma cortisol after 1 mg dexamethasone at bedtime | Urinary cortisol after variable doses of dexamethasone, adrenal CT and scintiscans |
| Pheochromocytoma | Spot urine for metanephrine | Urinary catechols; plasma catechols (basal and after 0.3 mg clonidine) Adrenal CT and scintiscans |

*Table 8*
*Overall guide to workup for secondary causes of hypertension*

elsewhere. If the initial screening studies are positive, the additional studies should be obtained.

If identifiable causes seem unlikely on the basis of the history, physical examination and routine laboratory work, the next step is to begin treatment. The evidence that such treatment is beneficial for the elderly with hypertension is examined next.

**Age of onset: <20 or >50**

**Level of blood pressure >180/110 mmHg**

**Organ damage**

  Funduscopy grade II or beyond
  Serum creatinine > 1.5 mg/dl
  Cardiomegaly or left ventricular hypertrophy as
    determined by electrocardiography

**Presence of features indicative of secondary causes**

  Unprovoked hypokalaemia
  Abdominal bruit
  Variable pressures with tachycardia, sweating,
    tremor
  Family history of renal disease

**Poor response to generally affective therapy**

*Table 9*
*Features of 'inappropriate' hypertension*

## The benefits of treating hypertension in the elderly

Over the past few years, increasingly strong evidence from large randomized controlled trials (RCTs) has documented the value of treating hypertension in the elderly. As shown by MacMahon and Rodgers (1993) (Figure 23), the protection against stroke, a 34% decrease, and coronary heart disease (CHD), a 19% decrease, in the five RCTs completed prior to 1997 in elderly patients is quantitatively greater than that shown in multiple RCTs in younger subjects. In particular, the reduction in CHD was almost twice that seen in the younger patients which is probably a reflection of two factors.

- The elderly start at a much higher risk than the younger and therefore are more likely to achieve benefit over the relatively short time, ie, 4–6 years, of these RCTs. If younger patients were treated for 10–20 years, they would almost certainly achieve as much benefit.

- Therapy in the more recent RCTs in the elderly was based on low doses of diuretic which are clearly more cardioprotective than the higher

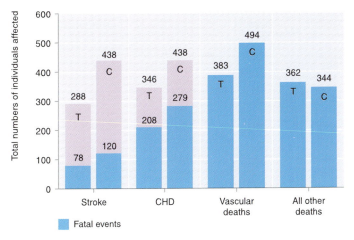

**Figure 23**

*Effects of blood pressure reduction on stroke and CHD events, vascular death, and non-vascular death in elderly patients. Combined results of five randomized trials of antihypertensive treatments in patients >60 years old. Data for 12 483 patients; SBP difference 12–14 mmHg; DBP difference 5–6 mmHg; follow-up, 5 years. Percent reduction in odds: 34% (SD = 6; P<0.0001) for stroke; 19% (7 SD; P<0.05) for CHD; 23% (6 SD; P<0.001) for vascular deaths; -7% (8 SD; P>0.5) for all other deaths. T, treatment; C, contol. (From MacMahon and Rodgers 1993.)*

doses of diuretic used in the earlier RCTs in younger patients. As shown by Psaty et al (1997) (Figure 24) both low doses (up to 25 mg of hydrochlorothiazide or its equivalent) and high doses (50 mg and more) of diuretic provided protection against stoke, as did beta-blocker based therapy. For CHD, however, only low-dose diuretic based therapy has been beneficial.

| Outcome drug regimen | Dose | No. of trials | Events, active treatment/ control | RR (95% CI) |
|---|---|---|---|---|
| Stroke | | | | |
| Diuretics | High | 9 | 88/232 | 0.49 (0.39-0.62) |
| Diuretics | Low | 4 | 191/347 | 0.66 (0.55-0.78) |
| β-blockers | | 4 | 147/335 | 0.71 (0.59-0.86) |
| HDFP | High | 1 | 102/158 | 0.64 (0.50-0.82) |
| Coronary heart disease | | | | |
| Diuretics | High | 11 | 211/331 | 0.99 (0.83-1.18) |
| Diuretics | Low | 4 | 215/363 | 0.72 (0.61-0.85) |
| β-blockers | | 4 | 243/459 | 0.93 (0.80-1.09) |
| HDFP | High | 1 | 171/189 | 0.90 (0.73-1.10) |

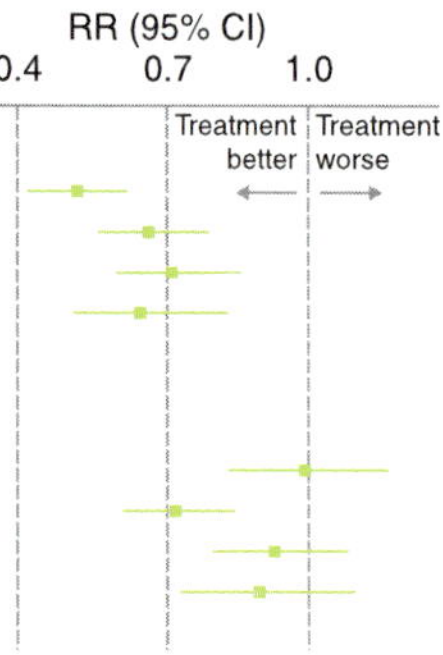


***Figure 24***
*Meta-analysis of randomized, placebo-controlled clinical trials in hypertension according to first-line treatment strategy. For these comparisons, the number of participants randomized to active therapy and placebo were 7758 and 12 075 for high-dose diuretic therapy; 4305 and 5116 for low-dose diuretic therapy; and 6736 and 12 147 for beta-blocker therapy. RR, relative risk; CI, confidence interval. (From Psaty et al 1997.)*

As will be noted, one additional RCT in the elderly has been published, the Syst-Eur trial reported by Staessen et al (1997). The trial used a long-acting dihydropyridine calcium antagonist, nitrendipine, the first RCT to use any drug other than a diuretic or beta-blocker.

In view of the importance of these recent RCTs, each will be highlighted. They, along with the data from prior RCTs involving smaller numbers of elderly hypertensives, provide unequivocal evidence that treatment reduces cardiovascular morbidity and mortality (Mulrow et al 1994) (Figure 25). Note the small number of elderly patients needed to be treated for 5 years (5y-NNT) to prevent one patient from having a cardiovascular event or from dying from cardiovascular disease.

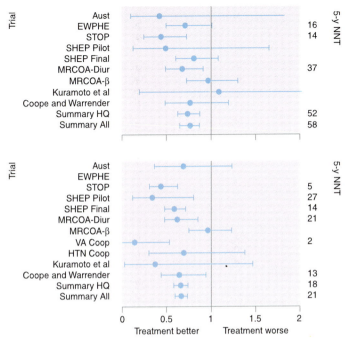

**Figure 25**

*Quantitative analyses of recent, large, placebo-controlled, high-quality trials presented at odds ratios with 95% confidence intervals. Summary results are presented for elderly recent high-quality (HQ) trials and for all trials. Aust, Australian National Blood Pressure study; MRCOA-Dir, the diuretic arm of the Medical Research Council Trial in Older Adults; HTN Coop, Hypertension Detection and Follow-up Program Cooperative Group.*
*(From Mulrow et al 1994.)*

# The individual trials in the elderly

Tables 10–15 provide the important features of the major trials in the elderly. A bit more about the Syst-Eur trial will be provided since it is different in a critical way from the others.

| | |
|---|---|
| **Number of subjects** | 840 |
| **Age group** | 60+ (mean age 72) |
| **Treatment tested** | Hydrochlorothiazide and triamterene versus placebo |
| **Study design** | Recruited from outpatient clinics double blind, randomized, followed up for 4.5 years |
| **Blood pressure criteria** | >160/90 mmHg |
| **Results** | Significant reduction in cardiovascular mortality and deaths from myocardial infarction |
| | Non-significant reduction in cerebrovascular deaths and overall mortality |
| | Main benefits seen in those aged less than 80 years and with moderate reduction in blood pressure |

**Table 10**
*European Working Party on Hypertension in the Elderly (EWHPE) Trial (From Amery et al 1985.)*

| | |
|---|---|
| **Number of subjects** | 840 |
| **Age group** | 60–79 |
| **Treatment tested** | *Atenolol + bendrofluazide versus placebo* |
| **Study design** | Recruited from general practices followed up for 4.5 years |
| **Blood pressure criteria** | >170/105 mmHg |
| **Results** | • Significant reduction in fatal and total strokes |
| | • Non-significant reduction in cardiovascular mortality |
| | • No effect on incidence of myocardial infarction |

*Table 11*
Hypertension Elderly Patients (HPE) Trial
(from Coope and Warrender 1986.)

| | |
|---|---|
| **Number of subjects** | 4736 |
| **Age group** | > 60(mean age 72) |
| **Treatment tested** | Chorthalidone versus placebo (chorthalidone switched to atenolol or reserpine if ineffective) |
| **Study design** | Double blind, randomized followed for 5 years |
| **Blood pressure criteria** | Systolic >160 mmHg Diastolic < 90 mmHg |
| **Results** | • Significant reductions in: <br>  −stroke incidence <br>  −myocardial infarction incidence <br>  −cardiovascular deaths <br>  −cardiovascular events <br>  −overall mortality <br> • Equal benefit seen in those aged over 80 as well as under 80 years |

*Table 12*
*Systolic Hypertension in the Elderly Project (SHEP)*
*(From SHEP Cooperative Research Group 1991.)*

| | |
|---|---|
| **Number of subjects** | 1627 |
| **Age group** | 70–84 |
| **Treatment tested** | Thiazide versus β-blockers versus placebo |
| **Study design** | Double blind, randomized followed for 25 months |
| **Blood pressure criteria** | Systolic >180 mmHg diastolic 90–110 mmHg |
| **Results** | • Significant reductions in:<br>–fatal and non-fatal strokes<br>–cardiovascular events<br>–cardiovascular and total mortality<br>• Non-significant reduction in incidence of myocardial infarction |

*Table 13*
*Swedish Trial in Old Patients with Hypertension (STOP–HT)*
*(From Dahlof et al 1991.)*

| | |
|---|---|
| **Number of subjects** | 4396 |
| **Age group** | 65–75 |
| **Treatment tested** | Atenolol versus hydrochlorothiazide plus amiloride versus placebo |
| **Study design** | Single blind, randomized |
| **Blood pressure criteria** | Systolic >180 mmHg Diastolic 90–110 mmHg |
| **Results** | • Significant reductions in: <br> –stroke <br> –cardiovascular events <br> –coronary events <br> only in the diuretic group <br> • Non-significant reduction in end-points seen with atenolol |

**Table 14**
*Medical Research Council trial of treatment of hypertension in older adults (From MRC Working Party 1992.)*

| Number of subjects | 4695 |
|---|---|
| Age group | 60+ (mean age 70) |
| Treatment tested | Nitrendipine; possible addition of enalapril and hydrochlorothiazide versus placebo |
| Study design | Recruited from 198 centres in 23 European countries<br>Double blind, randomized; followed for up to 7 years (median 24 month) |
| Blood pressure criteria | Systolic 160–219 mmHg<br>Diastolic <95 mmHg |
| Results | • Significant reduction in:<br>–fatal and non-fatal strokes (42%)<br>–fatal and non-fatal cardiac events (26%)<br>• Non-significant reductions in myocardial infarction (30%) and heart failure (29%) |

*Table 15*
Systolic hypertension in Europe (Sys-Eur) trial
(From Staessen et al 1997.)

## The Syst-Eur trial (Figure 26)

As of late 1998, this is the only RCT in the elderly to be reported in which any drug other than diuretics or beta-blockers were used. As will be noted later, this RCT also provides another piece of evidence that lowering the blood pressure of elderly hypertensives is beneficial. Until Syst-Eur, there was no definite evidence for any of the newer types of antihypertensive agents including ACE inhibitors, alpha-blockers and calcium antagonists.

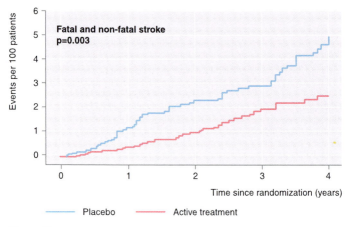

*Figure 26*
*Cumulative rates of fatal and non-fatal stroke in the placebo and active treatment groups in the SYST-Eur trial. (From Staessen et al, 1997.)*

It is likely that Syst-Eur and two additional trials from China are the last to be placebo-controlled, since it is no longer considered ethical to leave hypertensives, young or old, on placebo for more than a few months. A large number of trials are in the process of comparing different drugs against each other, including the massive ALLHAT (Antihypertensive and Lipid Lowering Heart Attack Prevention Trial) study now in progress in the United States.

## The STONE trial

One additional trial in the elderly has been published by Gong et al (1996), the Shanghai Trial of Nifedipine in the Elderly (STONE). The patients in this trial were entered sequentially and not randomly into the active or placebo groups, thereby giving rise to possible bias. Nonetheless, the data are quite consistent with the other trials in the elderly, showing significant reductions in stroke and overall mortality with nifedipine tablets (15 deaths in 817 patients) compared to placebo (26 deaths in 815 patients).

Data from another RCT from China, the Syst-China trial, was presented in mid-1998 and will probably be published soon. The design of Syst-China was virtually identical to the Syst-Eur trial and the results appear to be virtually identical: significant reductions in stroke and cardiac events with the long-acting dihydropyridine calcium antagonist nitrendipine compared to placebo in elderly hypertensives.

## *Beta-blocker based trials*

As noted in the Joint National Committee report (JNC-6) but even more definitively shown by Messerli et al (1998) (Figure 27), the results of the two RCTs in the elderly in which therapy was based on a beta-blocker did not show a reduction in coronary events or overall cardiovascular mortality. There are numerous potential reasons for this inadequacy as detailed by Messerli et al. As will be noted later, beta-blockers are useful drugs in some elderly patients but, as recommended in JNC-6, they should always be combined with a diuretic for treatment of hypertension since only such combinations have been shown to be beneficial in the treatment of hypertension in the elderly.

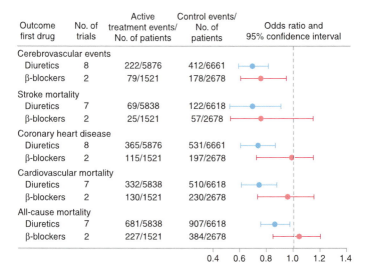

| Outcome first drug | No. of trials | Active treatment events/ No. of patients | Control events/ No. of patients | Odds ratio and 95% confidence interval |
|---|---|---|---|---|
| **Cerebrovascular events** | | | | |
| Diuretics | 8 | 222/5876 | 412/6661 | |
| β-blockers | 2 | 79/1521 | 178/2678 | |
| **Stroke mortality** | | | | |
| Diuretics | 7 | 69/5838 | 122/6618 | |
| β-blockers | 2 | 25/1521 | 57/2678 | |
| **Coronary heart disease** | | | | |
| Diuretics | 8 | 365/5876 | 531/6661 | |
| β-blockers | 2 | 115/1521 | 197/2678 | |
| **Cardiovascular mortality** | | | | |
| Diuretics | 7 | 332/5838 | 510/6618 | |
| β-blockers | 2 | 130/1521 | 230/2678 | |
| **All-cause mortality** | | | | |
| Diuretics | 7 | 681/5838 | 907/6618 | |
| β-blockers | 2 | 227/1521 | 384/2678 | |

*Figure 27*
*Outcome of various end-points in 7 or 8 trials in the elderly using a diuretic or in 2 trials using a beta-blocker as first drug. (From Messerli et al, 1998.)*

# When should therapy be started?

In the past, guidelines for the institution of therapy have been based solely on the level of blood pressure, giving rise to major irrationalities and inconsistencies. As noted by Jackson et al (1993):

'This has led to the situation in which a 60 year old woman with a DBP of 100 mmHg but no other risk factors (her absolute risk of cardiovascular disease is about 10% in 10 years) may meet the criteria for treatment, whereas a 70 year old man with multiple risk factors but a DBP of 95 mmHg (his absolute risk is about 50% in 10 years) may not'.

On the basis of the results of the multiple clinical trials wherein reductions of blood pressure by about 10/5 mmHg resulted in reductions of overall cardiovascular risk by about one-third, the treatment of these two patients would be expected to reduce the absolute risk in the 60-year-old woman by about 3% in 10 years (30% of 10%) but in the 70-year-old man by about 17% (30% of 50%). As Jackson et al (1993) note:

'In other words, if 100 women aged 60 with DBP of 100 mmHg and no other risk factors were treated for 10 years, about 3 events would be prevented, whereas if 100 men aged 70 with a DBP of 95 mmHg and multiple other risk factors were treated, about 17 events would be prevented'.

Fortunately, there is now widespread recognition of the need to consider numerous factors beyond just the level of blood pressure in making the decision to treat. JNC-6 provides criteria for three risk groups, based on the level of blood pressure, the presence of major risk factors, such as target organ damage or clinical cardiovascular disease (Table 16). It is recommended to start management of the three risk groups with either lifestyle modification alone or with drug therapy (Table 17).

Age, in itself, (over 60 years) is one major risk factor and most of the elderly with hypertension will have systolics above 160 mmHg so that immediate drug therapy will be indicated for a large proportion of the elderly. Nonetheless, as we shall see later, lifestyle modifications certainly have an important role in the management of the elderly hypertensive.

| Characteristics | Risk group A | Risk group B | Risk group C |
|---|---|---|---|
| Major risk factors | – | + | –/+ |
| Target organ damage or clinical cardiovascular disease | – | – | + |
| **Blood pressure mmHg (stages)** | | | |
| 130–139/85–89 (high–normal) | Lifestyle modification | Lifestyle modification | Drug therapy§ |
| 140–159/90–99 (stage 1) | Lifestyle modification (up to 12 months) | Lifestyle modification‡ (up to 6 months) | Drug therapy |
| ≤160/ ≥100 (stages 2 and 3) | Drug therapy | Drug therapy | Drug therapy |

Modified from Joint National Committee 1997
  Minus sign, absent; plus sign, present.
* Lifestyle modification should be adjunctive
  therapy for all patients recommended for pharmacological therapy.
§ For those with heart failure, renal failure, or diabetes.
‡ For patients with multiple risk factors, clinicians should consider drugs as initial
  therapy plus lifestyle modifications.

**Table 16**
*Risk stratification and treatment*

## Is there an age limit for therapy?

None of the RCTs in the elderly included enough patients over the age of 80 to determine the value of antihypertensive therapy in such patients, the most rapidly growing part of our population. Until trials now in progress provide definite evidence, the best course is to treat – ever so gently – very old patients with systolic blood pressure above 160 mmHg or diastolic blood pressure above 90 mmHg if they seem likely to have more than 1 year of life survival. Those who are severely debilitated with end-stage cancer or dementia are best left untreated. However, a 100-year-old who can be protected from stroke or dementia and thereby

*Table 17*
*Components of cardiovascular risk stratification in patients with hypertension*

allowed to maintain an enjoyable life should not be denied such benefit.

Furthermore, there seems no reason to stop successful and well tolerated therapy, regardless of the attained age. As will be noted later, almost all who are hypertensive before treatment will become hypertensive again if treatment is stopped. If blood pressure becomes lower than 140/85 mmHg, treatment logically should be reduced so as not to keep blood pressure below the level needed for adequate tissue perfusion.

# The goal of therapy

Perhaps the issue of how far to reduce the blood pressure should come after the details on therapy but establishing the goal of therapy is an essential aspect of treatment and should be established 'up front'.

There are three possible relationships between the levels of blood pressure achieved by therapy and the risk of cardio-vascular disease (Figure 28). Line A implies the lower the blood pressure, the less the risk, in keeping with the straight-line relationship between untreated levels of blood pressure and risk shown in Figure 10. However, the results of the multiple RCTs described earlier have suggested that the consequences of therapy are more accurately por-trayed as either line B, wherein little if any additional bene-fit is derived from increasingly greater reduction in blood pressure, or line C, wherein additional risks appear as the pressure is reduced below some initial level. As is obvious, line C delineates a 'J-curve', the term used for the third scenario.

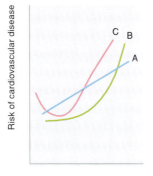

**Figure 28**
*Three models of hypothetical relationships between levels of blood pressure and risk of cardiovascular disease. (From Epstein 1980.)*

From the time in 1979 when the English practitioner I.M.G. Stewart reported a five-fold increase in heart attacks among patients whose diastolic blood pressure (4th Korotkoff phase) was reduced below 90 mmHg, considerable arguments have both defended and denied the presence of a J-curve. The reason why so much discussion has been held is the implication that therapy beyond a certain level could have serious adverse consequences.

The massive Hypertension Optimal Treatment (HOT) trial (Hanson et al 1998) was designed primarily to answer the issue in a prospective manner, since most of the data for and against the J-curve were retrospective analyses of small numbers of patients. The HOT trial involved almost 19 000 hypertensives aged 50–80 years old (mean 61.5 years) with diastolic blood pressure between 100 and 115 mmHg while on no therapy. They were randomly divided into three groups to receive drug therapy adequate to lower their diastolic blood pressure to either 90, 85 or 80 mmHg. Therapy began with the long-acting dihydropyridine calcium antagonist, felodipine, and other drugs (ACE inhibitor, beta-blocker, diuretic) could be added to achieve the target blood pressure.

Unfortunately, at the end of the average 3.8 year follow-up, the separation between the three groups was less than half of the 10 mmHg desired. Therefore, the existence of a J-curve could be neither denied nor documented because of the small degree of blood pressure differences. Nonetheless, when all of the data were analysed, the relation between achieved blood pressure and cardiovascular risk did show that the 'best' blood pressure with the minimum number of major adverse events was 138.5/82.6 mmHg (Figure 29). No additional benefit was seen at lower blood pressure. The authors of the HOT trial paper provide arguments against the J-curve. However, a closer look at Figure 29 show a rise, slight but definite, in cardiovascular events and mortality at diastolic blood pressure below 85 mmHg.

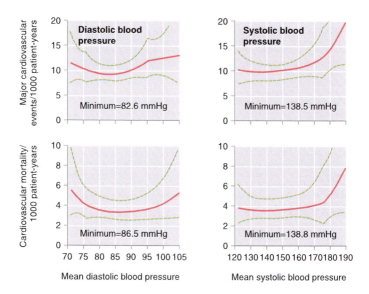

**Figure 29**

*Estimated incidence with 95% confidence interval of major cardiovascular events (top) and cardiovascular mortality (bottom) in relation to achieved mean diastolic and systolic blood pressure in the HOT trial.*
*(From Hansson et al 1998.)*

To this author, the J-curve continues to be likely for coronary events. However for stroke and even more certainly for progressive renal damage, 'the lower the better' seems to be true. Moreover, the 1500 high-risk diabetic hypertensives in the HOT trial did better with the lowest blood pressures achieved, documenting further the need for more intensive therapy for this vulnerable population.

We are left, then, with a goal of 140/85 mmHg for most patients and lower goals, still uncertain as to the level, for higher risk patients including those with diabetes or renal damage. Based upon the HOT trial and the previously described RCTs in the elderly, a systolic blood pressure of 140 mmHg seems appropriate for the elderly with isolated systolic hypertensive. Even though their already low diastolic blood pressure may go down further, no apparent trouble was seen with such low diastolic levels at an average of 69 mmHg in the Systolic Hypertension in the Elderly (SHEP 1991) trial. If postural hypotension or other symptoms of decreased blood flow are noted, a decrease in the lowering of systolic blood pressure may be appropriate.

Now that the goal of therapy is defined, we will see how best to accomplish that goal, starting with lifestyle modifications, also known as non-drug therapy.

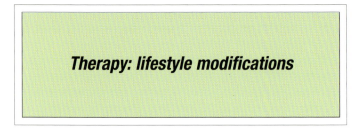

# *Therapy: lifestyle modifications*

A number of lifestyle changes are known to lower blood pressure in a significant portion of the hypertensive population (Joint National Commitee 1997) (Table 18). Not all of these have been studied in elderly patients but their benefits almost certainly apply to them equally as much or even more. For instance, elderly people respond more to a lower sodium intake, ie, they are more sodium sensitive as noted earlier (Figure 4).

Stop smoking
Lose weight if overweight
Limit alcohol intake to $\leq$1ounce/day of ethanol
   (24 ounces of beer, 8 ounces of wine, or 2 ounces
   of 100-proof whiskey)
Reduce sodium intake to 110 mmol/day (2.4 g
   sodium or 6 g sodium chloride)
Maintain adequate dietary potassium, calcium, and
   magnesium intake
Reduce dietary saturated fat and cholesterol intake
   for overall cardiovascular health
Exercise (aerobic) regularly

**Table 18**
*Lifestyle modifications for hypertension*

# Avoidance of tobacco

Nicotine has an acute and often dramatic pressor effect that does not lessen with continued exposure. Tolerance to many of the other noxious effects of nicotine develops, but the rise in blood pressure occurs with every exposure (Groppelli et al 1992) (Figure 30). The pressor effect noted in these addicted smokers from the cigarette smoked for 2 min persisted for approximately 15 min as shown in Figure 30. Therefore the effect may not be recognized since smoking is not allowed in clinics or offices where blood pressure is measured. The time from the last puff in the parking lot to the measurement of blood pressure may be far greater than the duration of the last puff's pressor effect. Therefore, smokers should take their blood pressure while smoking. That blood pressure should be the basis for deciding upon therapy and the goal of therapy. Regardless of age or duration of smoking, every effort should be made to get the patient to stop.

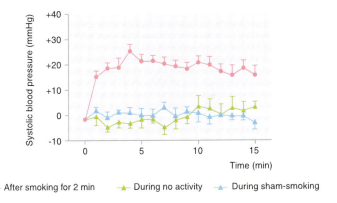

— After smoking for 2 min      — During no activity      — During sham-smoking

**Figure 30**
*Changes in systolic blood pressure over 15 min after smoking the first cigarette of the day in 10 normotensive smokers.*
*(From Groppelli et al 1992.)*

# Weight loss

Weight gain is the most common direct environmental cause of hypertension. Even relatively small amounts of weight gain increase the incidence of hypertension as shown in the report by Huang et al (1998) of a 20 year follow-up of 82 000 US nurses. Those who gained as little as 5 kg (11 lb) from their weight at age 18 had twice as much hypertension as those whose weight did not change; with a 10 kg (22 lb) weight gain, the incidence tripled. The effect was less in the women who were now over the age of 55 than in those younger but these data clearly indicate the major contribution of even modest weight gain on the risk for hypertension.

Furthermore, those who lost weight had less hypertension, in keeping with a large body of data showing falls in blood pressure with weight loss (Figure 31). As difficult as it may be, particularly for the elderly, weight loss must be constantly urged upon all overweight hypertensives and they should be given appropriate dietary advice. Short-term use of diet pills may be of some help but caution is needed since most can raise blood pressure.

# Sodium restriction

Despite a seriously flawed claim by Alderman et al (1998) that coronary risk was increased among those who ingested a low sodium diet, the evidence is overwhelming that modest sodium restriction is both safe and effective in lowering blood pressure. Numerous meta-analyses of controlled trials have shown a small but significant and almost uniform lowering of blood pressure by a 40–60 mmol/day reduction in sodium intake, approximating the usual recommendation of a 100–110 mmol/day intake.

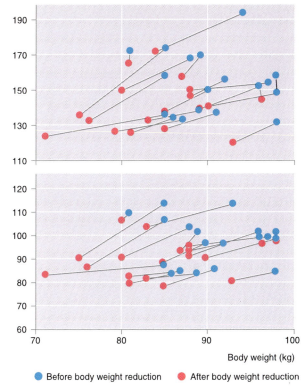

*Figure 31*
*Systolic and diastolic blood pressure before and after body weight reduction.*
*(From Staessen et al 1989.)*

The elderly are more sodium sensitive and therefore are more likely to respond favorably to sodium restriction. Two factors may make it more difficult for them to restrict sodium: first, taste sensation may diminish with age so more salt may be added to achieve the desired degree of saltiness; second, the elderly may be more dependent on processed and packaged foods which usually have large amounts of sodium added (Table 19).

| Higher sodium (mg/serving) | |
| --- | --- |
| Hunt's whole tomatoes | 660 |
| Rice-A-Roni | 520 |
| Del Monte whole kernel corn | 360 |
| Kraft American cheese | 450 |
| Kellogg's cornflakes | 290 |
| Pace chunky salsa | 359 |
| Oscar Mayer turkey | 687 |

| Lower sodium (mg/serving) | |
| --- | --- |
| Tomatoes, fresh | 16 |
| Rice, enriched white | 3 |
| Corn, fresh | 14 |
| Kraft Cheddar cheese | 180 |
| Nabisco shredded wheat | 0 |
| Enrico chunky salsa | 75 |
| Tyson turkey breast | 272 |

Data from food labels and the US Department of Agriculture, Composition of Foods, Raw, Processed, Prepared (Handbook 8)

*Table 19*
*Sodium in equal amounts of differently processed foods*

The effort is worthwhile and, with counselling, avoidance of processed foods with more than 300 mg of sodium per portion as indicated on the label (a major boon to sodium avoidance), and occasional checks of urinary sodium excretion, success can be achieved.

## The TONE trial

Perhaps the best documentation of the benefits and safety of modest sodium restriction, alone or combined with weight loss, in elderly hypertensives comes from the randomized controlled Trial of Nonpharmacologic Interventions in the Elderly (TONE) reported by Whelton et al (1998) (Figure 32). The trial involved men and women aged 60–80 years with hypertension that was being well controlled on one or two medications. The patients agreed to discontinue their drugs and were then randomly allocated to four groups: (1) no changes, ie, usual care; (2) modest dietary sodium restriction; (3) weight loss by caloric restriction and increased physical activity; and (4) both sodium restriction and weight loss. Over a 30 month follow-up, the patients achieved only modest reductions in sodium intake (an average of 40 mmol/day) and weight loss (an average of 4.7 kg or 10.3 lbs). Despite these modest changes, the number whose hypertension reappeared (the primary end-point) and who developed cardiovascular complications was far greater among the usual care group than among those who reduced either sodium intake or body weight. Those who did both were protected even more.

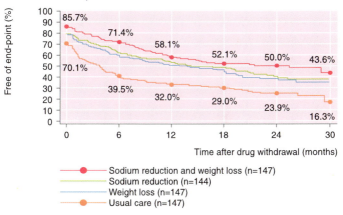

**Figure 32**
*Percentage of the participants assigned to both sodium restriction and weight loss, to sodium restriction alone, to weight loss alone, and to usual care (no intervention) who remained free of cardiovascular events and recurrence of hypertension during the 30 month follow-up of the TONE study. (From Whelton et al 1988.)*

The TONE data are particularly meaningful because the trial involved elderly hypertensives, it went on for 30 months, and it documented the benefits of only modest lifestyle changes which should be achievable in the 'real world'. Such prospective controlled observations, moreover, give a much more accurate view of the potential risks of these manoeuvres than retrospective, uncontrolled observations such as those by Alderman and co-workers.

## *Limit alcohol intake*

Too much alcohol raises blood pressure (Figure 33); too little increases coronary risk. The appropriate amount, ie, one-half portion/day for women and up to two portions/day for men, does not raise the blood pressure but does provide protection from coronary mortality. (A portion contains 10–12 ml of ethanol = 1.5 ounces of 100 proof spirits, 4 ounces of wine, 12 ounces of beer).

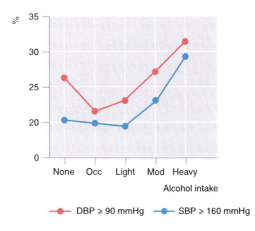

**Figure 33**
*Age-adjusted prevalence rates (in percent) of measured systolic and diastolic hypertension by levels of alcohol intake in drinks. Occ, occasional; light, one to two daily; Mod, moderate, three to six daily; Heavy, more than six daily. (From Shaper et al 1988.)*

Too much alcohol is probably the most common cause of easily reversible hypertension, the estimate being 8% of hypertensive men in the US (Kaplan 1998). Those who drink more than 2 portions on average per day must be strongly advised to cut back.

Small amounts of daily alcohol consumption protect against coronary mortality as shown in multiple surveys including that of Thun et al (1997) who followed 490 000 men and women for 9 years after ascertainment of their alcohol use. All-cause and cardiovascular mortality was reduced by 30–40% in those who drank at least one drink daily compared to those who did not drink. As expected, mortality from alcohol-related diseases increased with excessive consumption.

The lower recommendation for women should circumvent any threat of stimulation of breast cancer by alcohol.

## Maintain adequate dietary potassium, calcium and magnesium

Intake of these three minerals should be well maintained in the elderly, if not by the diet containing adequate amounts of fresh fruits, vegetables and dairy products then by mineral and vitamin supplements.

Increased intake of 40–80 mmol/day of potassium, preferably in fresh fruits and vegetables, will lower blood pressure almost as much as will moderate sodium restriction. On the other hand, as reviewed by Sachs et al (1998), increased intake of calcium or magnesium will not affect blood pressure even in those with low habitual intakes.

# Exercise regularly

Of the entire 'lifestyle prescription', regular physical activity may be the most difficult to accomplish in this world of 'couch potatoes' but the one that will provide the most benefit. As shown by Hakim et al (1998) in their study of older physically capable men, regular walking reduced overall mortality. The longer the walk, the lower the mortality.

Such low intensity activity will also lower blood pressure which will probably contribute to the overall reduction in mortality. Higher intensity activity may be even better, both to aid in weight loss and to lower blood pressure. Pure isometric exercise (weightlifting) only raises blood pressure acutely; during aerobic or isotonic activity (running, swimming) systolic blood pressure increases and diastolic goes down. Afterwards both systolic and diastolic levels tend to remain lower.

Those elderly hypertensives who cannot walk, run or swim should be encouraged to use whatever exercise devices they can that are available at health clubs and retirement centres.

# Reduce dietary saturated fat and cholesterol

There is very likely some benefit upon the blood pressure when serum lipids are lowered by diet or statin drug therapy. The effect is mediated by improvements in endothelial function with increased synthesis of vasodilatory nitric oxide. In most trials of lipid-lowering agents, a slight but significant fall in blood pressure has been observed as summarized by Goode et al (1995).

# Other modalities

Increased amounts of fibre, omega-3 fatty acids, garlic or oral antioxidants as well as various relaxation techniques have been claimed to lower blood pressure but most of the trials are small, short and poorly controlled (Kaplan 1998). None of these should have adverse effects but do not expect them to lower blood pressure.

Two additional drugs are widely used among elderly hypertensives: aspirin and oestrogens as replacement therapy (ORT). Aspirin, 75 mg daily was shown in the HOT trial to reduce coronary events but to increase non-fatal bleeding episodes. ORT, unlike oral contraceptives, does not raise blood pressure and can be given to hypertensive women without concern about their blood pressure.

After these lifestyle changes have been attempted, the blood pressure may remain above the goal, making drug therapy compulsory.

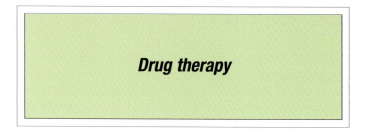

# Drug therapy

Treatment of hypertension in the elderly differs in a number of both obvious and subtle ways from the treatment of younger patients. In part as a reflection of the different pathophysiology described earlier but mainly because of the multiple 'natural' changes occurring with age, the elderly need to be treated cautiously, following the admonition: 'start low and go slow'.

Since the elderly may have sluggish baroreceptor and sympathetic nervous responsiveness as well as impaired cerebral autoregulation, therapy should be gentle and gradual, avoiding drugs that are likely to cause postural hypotension or to exacerbate other common problems often seen among the elderly (Table 20). Even more caution is advised with the very old. Langer et al (1993) observed an increase in mortality over 5 years among 400 men over the age of 75 whose diastolic blood pressure was reduced by 5 mmHg or more by antihypertensive therapy.

These cautions should not, however, interfere with the well documented need to treat the overwhelming majority of elderly hypertensives. The benefits they have been shown to receive from antihypertensive drug therapy detailed earlier are quantitatively greater than provided to younger

| Factors | Potential complications |
| --- | --- |
| Diminished baroreceptor activity | Orthostatic hypotension |
| Impaired cerebral autoregulation | Cerebral ischaemia with small falls in systemic pressure |
| Decreased intravascular volume | Orthostatic hypotension |
| Sensitivity to hypokalaemia | Volume depletion, hyponatraemia |
| Decreased renal and hepatic function | Arrhythmia, muscular weakness |
| Polypharmacy | Drug accumulation |
| CNS changes | Drug interactions |
|  | Depression, confusion |

**Table 20**
*Factors that might contribute to increased risk of pharmacological treatment of hypertension in the elderly*

patients. No longer should age alone interfere with the provision of appropriate therapy.

# General guidelines

The treatment algorithm provided in the JNC-6 report (Joint National Comittee 1997) (Figure 34; Table 21) is well suited to the elderly hypertensive, with the caveat that few will have 'uncomplicated' hypertension and more will have one or more of the compelling and specific indications listed in Table 21. Since the majority will have isolated systolic hypertension, attention will be directed to the compelling indications for diuretics as the preferred initial therapy and the use of long-acting dihydropyridine (DHP) calcium antagonists as an appropriate alternative.

### Diuretics for initial therapy

As shown earlier, a low dose of a diuretic was the first drug used in all but one of the six major randomized controlled trials (RCTs) in the elderly. In the MRC Trial, half of those allocated to drug therapy received the beta-blocker atenolol. A large amount of data from the Systolic Hypertension in the Elderly (SHEP) trial has confirmed the efficacy and safety of the step 1 drug, chlorthalidone, started at 12.5 mg/day and increased if needed to 25 mg/day. As reported by Savage et al (1998), this low-dose diuretic regimen was well tolerated and effective in reducing blood pressure by 13/4 mmHg below that noted in the placebo-treated half. Biochemical changes were relatively minimal over the 3 years of active therapy (Table 22). New onset of diabetes occurred in 8.6% of diuretic treated compared to 7.5% of the placebo group.

In a substudy of the SHEP trial reported by Ofili et al (1998), the low-dose diuretic regimen induced a significant 13% reduction in left ventricular mass as assessed by echocardiography while a 6% increase in left ventricular mass was noted in the placebo group over the 3 year follow-up.

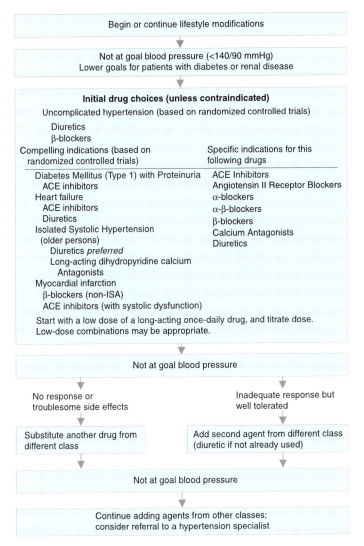

**Figure 34**
*The JNC-6 treatment algorithm*

| Indication | Drug Therapy |
|---|---|
| **Compelling Indications Unless Contraindicated** | |
| Diabetes mellitus (type1) with proteinuria | ACE I |
| Heart failure | ACE I, diuretics |
| Isolated hypertension (older patients) | Diuretics (preferred), CA (long-acting DHP) |
| Myocardial infarction | β-blockers (non-ISA), ACE I with systolic dysfunction) |

| **May have Favourable Effects on Comorbid Conditions**† | |
|---|---|
| Angina | β-blockers, CA |
| Arterial tachycardia and fibrillation | β-blockers, CA (non-DHP) |
| Cyclosporine-induced hypertension (caution with the dose of cyclosporine) | CA |
| Diabetes mellitus (types 1 and 2) with proteinuria | ACE I (preferred), CA |
| Diabetes mellitus (type 2) | Low-dose diuretics |
| Dyslipidaemia | α-blockers |
| Essential tremor | β-blockers (non-CS) |
| Heart failure | Carvedilol, losartan potassium |
| Hyperthyroidism | β-blockers |
| Migraine | β-blockers (non-CS), CA (non-DHP) |
| Myocardial infarction | Diltiazem hydrochloride, verapamil hydrochloride |
| Osteoporosis | Thiazides |
| Preoperative hypertension | β-blockers |
| Prostatism (BPH) | α-blockers |
| Renal insufficiency (caution in renovascular hypertension and creatinine level >265.2 μmol/[>3 mg/dl] | ACE I |

**Table 21**
*Considerations for individualizing antihypertensive drug therapy*

These data along with those from the other RCTs described earlier strongly support the preference given to low-dose diuretics for the elderly. Emphasis should be given to the low

**May Have Unfavourable Effects on Comorbid Conditions†‡**

| | |
|---|---|
| Bronchospastic disease | β-blockers |
| Depression | β-blockers, central α-agonists, reserpine§ |
| Diabetes mellitus (types 1 and 2) | β-blockers, high-dose diuretics |
| Dyslipidaemia | β-blockers (non-ISA), diuretics (high dose) |
| Gout | Diuretics |
| 2° or 3° heart block | β-blockers,§ CA (non DHP)§ |
| Heart failure | β-blockers (except carvedilol), CA (except amlodipine besylate; felodipine) |
| Liver disease | Labetalol hydrochloride, methyldopa§ |
| Peripheral vascular disease | β-blockers |
| Pregnancy | ACE I,§ angiotensin II receptor blockers§ |
| Renal insufficiency | Potassium-sparing agents |
| Renovascular disease | ACE I, angiotensin II receptor blockers |

ACE I indicates angiotensin-converting enzyme inhibitors; BPH, benign prostatic hyperplasia; CA, calcium antagonists; DHP, dihydropyridine; ISA, intrinsic sympathomimetic activity; MI, myocardial infarction; and non-CS, noncardioselective.
†Conditions and drugs are listed in alphabetical order.
‡These drugs may be used with special monitoring unless contraindicated.
§Contraindicated.

doses, equivalent to 12.5 mg of hydrochlorothiazide used as initial therapy, an amount that provided adequate antihypertensive efficacy in about half of the participants.

| Active Treatment Compared to Placebo | | |
|---|---|---|
| Fasting glucose | +0.20 mmol/l | (+3.6 mg/dl) |
| Total cholesterol | +0.09 mmol/l | (+3.5 mg/dl) |
| HDL-cholesterol | -0.02 mmol/l | (-0.77 mg/dl) |
| Triglycerides | +0.9 mmol/l | (+17 mg/dl) |
| Creatinine | +2.8 µmol/l | (+0.03 mg/dl) |
| Uric acid | +35 µmol/l | (+0.06 mg/dl) |
| Potassium | -0.3 mmol/l | |

*Table 22*
*Changes in blood chemistries in the SHEP trial (data from Savage et al 1998)*

## Long-acting dihydropyridine calcium antagonists

As described earlier, three RCTs have been completed comparing one of these agents against placebo in elderly patients with isolated systolic hypertension (ISH). The two RCTs from China have seemingly had much less impact than the Syst-Eur trial reported by Staessen and co-workers. All three showed excellent protection from both stroke and coronary disease with either long-acting nitrendipine or nifedipine.

The cardioprotection provided by these long-acting DHP calcium antagonists should allay any concerns about the danger noted with very large doses of short-acting nifedipine in the highly vulnerable post-myocardial infarction period. As well documented by Grossman and Messerli (1997) and others, long-acting calcium antagonists do not abruptly lower blood pressure, thereby avoiding the activation of sympathetic activity that is seen with short-acting agents.

Another concern about short-acting calcium antagonists their promotion of cancer, as reported in retrospective uncontrolled observations has also been clearly documented not to apply to the long-acting agents. In the Syst-Eur trial (Staessen et al 1997), 15% less cancer was diagnosed in those on nitrendipine than in those on placebo. Multiple large surveys, including one involving over 16 000 patients reported by Rosenberg et al (1998), have documented the absence of any relation between calcium antagonists and cancer.

Since nitrendipine is not marketed in the US (or UK), the JNC-6 report considered the other long-acting DHP calcium antagonists that are available to be appropriate alternatives. These include amlodipine, felodipine, nifedipine XL or nisoldipine.

**Drugs for specific indications**

As seen in Table 21, a variety of comorbid conditions that are often seen in elderly hypertensives may be favourably influenced by one class of drugs or another, while others may be adversely affected by certain drugs. These individualized choices are based on clinical experience but they do not have the support of RCTs that would make their use 'compelling'. However, the wisdom of using an alpha-blocker to relieve the symptoms of prostatism while also lowering the blood pressure is obvious. As noted by Lieber (1998), alpha-blockade is now the accepted initial therapy for most patients with urinary obstructive symptoms, so only one drug will often manage the two conditions, hypertension and BPH which occur together in as many as 25 of elderly men.

ACE inhibitors and, if additional data document their equivalent efficacy, angiotensin II receptor blockers, are clearly indicated for diabetic hypertensives. If one of these agents is not sufficient to bring the blood pressure to below 130/80 mmHg a low dose of thiazide is the next logical step. If blood pressure is still too high, a calcium antagonist may be required.

Patients with renal insufficiency, defined as a serum creatinine above 1.5 mg/dl, almost always need a larger dose of more potent, loop diuretics to overcome the sodium retention that is largely responsible for the progressive hypertension seen with worsening renal function.

## *Special guidelines for the elderly*

These recommendations should be helpful in controlling hypertension in the elderly in addition to those described later that are aimed at improving compliance with therapy (Kaplan 1998).

1 Always check for postural hypotension before starting antihypertensive drug therapy to avoid even more precipitous falls in blood pressure. If present, utilize the various manoeuvres described earlier to overcome the postural falls in blood pressure.
2 Establish the goal of therapy as 140/85 mmHg or lower; those with coronary disease should not have their diastolics reduced below 80 mmHg; those with ISH should have their systolics reduced to 140 mmHg without concern about further lowering of diastolic blood pressure unless symptoms of tissue hypoperfusion appear; those with diabetes or renal insufficiency should have their blood pressure reduced below 130/80 mmHg.
3 Start with a low dose of a thiazide diuretic preferably in combination with a potassium-sparing agent; if the serum creatinine is above 1.5 mg/dl, metolazone once daily, multiple daily doses of furosemide or one or two daily doses of torsemide may be needed.

4 If the diuretic is inadequate or poorly tolerated, add or substitute a long-acting DHP calcium antagonist, again starting with a dose one-half the usual starting dose. Titrate slowly, every 4–8 weeks, until control is attained.

5 Use agents in addition to diuretics or DHP calcium antagonists that provide favourable influences on comorbid conditions as noted in Table 21.

6 If a beta-blocker is indicated, as with angina or post-myocardial infarction, always add a low dose of thiazide diuretic.

7 Always use once-a-day dosing with long-acting agents that provide full 24 h efficacy. Agents such as amlodipine and trandolapril with inherently longer durations of action are particularly attractive to cover the days when doses are skipped, a common occurrence.

8 Home monitoring of the blood pressure is extremely useful both to ensure adequate 24 h control by having early morning readings prior to the day's therapy and to avoid the office white-coat effect which may lead to inadvertent overtreatment. Office readings that are high because of the white-coat effect may cause the patient's hypertension to appear to be undertreated when it is, in fact, well controlled or even overtreated.

9 Avoid drug interactions which are more common in the elderly since they often take a number of different types of medication. As shown in Table 23 some potentiate antihypertensive efforts but the most common interaction is with non-steroidal anti-inflammatory agents (NSAIDs) which will antagonize the effects of all agents save calcium antagonists. As noted by Johnson (1998), about 15% of elderly hypertensives take a NSAID and antihypertensive drugs concurrently. Johnson recommends the use of physical therapy and other analgesics such as acetaminophen which do not interfere with antihypertensive drug efficacy.

Rochon and Gurwitz (1997) describe a 'prescribing cascade' in elderly patients which begins when NSAIDs raise the blood pressure so that antihypertensive therapy is begun, only to be antagonized by the NSAID, calling forth more antihypertensive therapy.

## The matter of impotence

Erectile impotence is common in elderly men, usually a consequence of atherosclerotic impingement of penile blood flow. Hypertension may add to the problem, which may be further aggravated by antihypertensive therapy. As reported by Grimm et al (1997), of the five classes of antihypertensives compared in the Treatment of Mild Hypertension Study (TOMHS), only diuretics significantly increased the incidence of erectile impotence. Only 15 mg of chlorthalidone was used so the problem can obviously be exacerbated by low doses of diuretic.

Until sildenafil (Viagra) became available, impotence that began after antihypertensive therapy was begun was usually best managed by stopping the drug(s) being given, waiting for the return of potency and re-starting therapy with a low dose of another class of drug. Now, the best course, if the antihypertensive therapy is otherwise effective and well tolerated, is to simply give Viagra which should have no interaction with any antihypertensive drug. Caution is obviously needed to avoid the use of Viagra with nitrates which may induce profound hypotension.

Even if all the guidelines are followed, compliance with therapy may be poor. Advice to improve compliance, is provided next.

## Drugs that potentiate antihypertensive effects

- Antipsychotic agents, especially phenthiazine
- Antidepressants, especially tricyclics
- L-dopa preparations
- Benzodiapezines
- Baclofen
- Alcohol

## Drugs that antagonize antihypertensive effects

- Corticosteroids
- Non-steroidal anti-inflammatory drugs

## Specific interactions leading to toxicity

*Thiazide diuretics*

| | |
|---|---|
| • Theophyllines, steroids or β-agonists | ↑risk of hypokalaemia ↓excretion |
| • Lithium | ↑risk of toxicity |
| • Carbamazepine | ↓risk of hyponatraemia |

*β-blockers*

| | |
|---|---|
| • Verapamil | Possible bradycardia, asystole, hypotension, heart failure |
| • Digoxin | Profound bradycardia |
| • Oral hypoglycaemics | Enhanced hypo-glycaemic effects, mask the warning signs of hypoglycaemia |

*Table 23*
*Drug interactions*

# Improving compliance

Fewer than half of patients begun on antihypertensive therapy will still be taking their medication after 1 year. According to a survey of over 1000 hypertensives in England reported by Jones et al (1995), the continuation rates at 6 months were between 40 and 50% regardless of the class of antihypertensive drug prescribed. On the other hand, Monane et al (1997) found better compliance with other classes than with diuretics among a group of 8600 elderly hypertensives enrolled in the New Jersey Medicare program from 1982 to 1988. Compliance worsened when multiple drugs were prescribed and improved with more physician visits.

Unfortunately, hypertension and its treatment fulfills many of the criteria that are known to reduce adherence to any therapy (Table 25). As an asymptomatic, chronic, incurable condition whose treatment requires daily therapy that may cause side effects and which provides no obvious benefit to the patient, it is easy to see why so few patients adhere closely to their therapy. Table 24 provides general guidelines to improve patient compliance. Unfortunately few of these have been documented to improve compliance to therapy. In their review of all published randomized trials of interventions to improve compliance, Haynes et al

Patient and disease characteristics
  Asymptomatic
  Chronic condition
  Condition suppressed, not cured
  No immediate consequences of stopping therapy
  Social isolation
  Disrupted home situation
  Psychiatric illness

Treatment characteristics
  Long duration of therapy
  Complicated regimens
  Expensive medications
  Side effects of medications
  Multiple behavioral modifications
  Lack of specific appointment times
  Long waiting time in office

**Table 24**
*Factors that reduce adherence to therapy*

(1996) could identify only 13 which meet their criteria for adequate study design. Five of these 13 RCTs of interventions versus control involved hypertensives. Improved adherence to antihypertensive therapy was noted with these interventions.

- One dose of drug/day compared to two doses/day
- Tailoring of therapy to individual patients
- Self-monitoring of pills and blood pressure
- Rewards for higher adherence and lower blood pressure
- Worksite care by nurses

These findings support the use of home blood pressure readings, simplified once-daily regimes that fit the individual patient's needs and easy access to convenient care. The elderly often have additional impediments to adherence to therapy, ranging from difficulty in opening child-proof containers to an inability to pay for expensive drugs to difficulty in reaching their health-care providers.

Hopefully, the guidelines provided in Table 25 and elsewhere in this book will help physicians and their patients to achieve the true goal of antihypertensive therapy: to control hypertension without adverse effects that interfere with the quality of life while providing protection from hypertension-induced cardiovascular morbidity and mortality.

Be aware of the problem and be alert to signs of patient non-adherence

Establish the goal of therapy: to reduce blood pressure to near normotensive levels with minimal or no side effects

Educate the patient about the disease and its treatment

Involve the patient in decision making
Encourage family support

Maintain contact with the patient

Encourage visits and calls to allied health personnel
Allow the pharmacist to monitor therapy
Give feedback to the patient via home BP readings
Make contact with patients who do not return

**Table 25**
*General guidelines to improve patient adherence to antihypertensive therapy*

Keep care inexpensive and simple

Do the least workup needed to rule out secondary causes
Obtain follow-up laboratory data only yearly unless indicated
more often
Use home blood pressure readings
Use non-drug, low cost therapies
Use once-daily doses of long-acting drugs
Use generic drugs and break larger doses of tablets in half
If appropriate, use combination tablets
Tailor medication to daily routines

Prescribe according to pharmacological principles

Add one drug at a time
Start with small doses, aiming for 5–10 mmHg reductions
at each step
Have medication taken immediately on awakening in the
morning or after 4 a.m. if patient awakens to void
Prevent volume overload with adequate diuretic and
sodium restriction

Be willing to stop unsuccessful therapy and try a different
approach

Anticipate side effects

Adjust therapy to ameliorate side effects that do not spontaneously disappear

Continue to add effective and tolerated drugs, stepwise, in
sufficient doses to achieve the goal of therapy

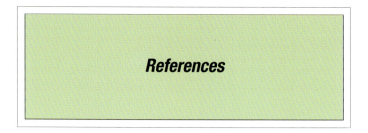

# References

Alderman MH, Cohen H, Madhavan S. Dietary sodium intake and mortality: the National health and nutrition examination survey (NHANES I). *Lancet* 1998; **351**:781–5.

Amery A, Brixko P, Clement D, et al. Mortality and morbidity results from the European Working Party in High Blood Pressure in the Elderly trial. *Lancet* 1985;**i**:1349–54.

Barker DJP. Fetal origins of coronary heart disease. *BMJ* 1995; **311**:171–4.

Boshuizen HC, Izaks GJ, van Buuren S, Ligthart GJ. Blood pressure and mortality in elderly people aged 85 and older: community based study. *BMJ* 1998; **316**:1780–4.

Brenner BM, Chertow GM. Congenital oligonephropathy and the etiology of adult hypertension and progressive renal injury. *Am J Kidney Dis* 1994; **23**:171–5.

British Hypertension Society. Technique of blood pressure meaurement. *Hypertension* 1995; **3**:293

Buck C, Baker P, Bass M, Donner A. The prognosis of hypertension according to age at onset. *Hypertension* 1987; **9**:204–8.

Burt VL, Whelton P, Roccella EJ et al. Prevalence of hypertension in the US adult population. Results from the Third National Health and Nutrition Examination Survey, 1988-91. *Hypertension* 1995;**25**:305–13.

Coope J, Warrender TS. Randomised trial of treatment of hypertension in elderly patients in primary care. *BMJ* 1986;**293**:1145–51

Dahlof B, Lindholm LH, Hansson L, et al. Morbidity and mortality in the Swedish Trial of Old Patients with Hypertension (STOP-Hypertension). *Lancet* 1991;**338**: 1281–85

Dodson PM, Lip GYH, Eames SM et al. Hypertensive retinopathy: a review of existing classification systems and a suggestion for a simplified grading system. *J Hum Hypertens* 1996; **10**:93–8.

Epstein FH. Primmary prevention of coronary heart disease. *Excerpta Medica* 1980; **i**:1–11

Forette FA, Seux ML, Thijs L, Staessen JA. Antihypertensive treatment and provention of dementia in older patients with isolated systolic hypertension: The SYST-EUR results. *J Hypertens* 1998; **16**:(Suppl 2) S22 [Abstract].

Gong L, Zhang W, Zhy Y et al. Shanghai trial of nifedipine in the elderly (STONE). *J Hypertens* 1996; **14**:1237-45.

Goode GK, Miller JP, Heagerty AM. Hyperlipidaemia, hypertension, and coronary heart disease. *Lancet* 1995; **345**:362–4.

Grimm RH, Grandits GA, Prineas RJ et al. Long-term effects on sexual function of five antihypertensive drugs and nutritional hygienic treatment in hypertensive men and women. *Hypertension* 1997; **29**:8–14.

Grodzicki T, Rajzer M, Fagard R et al. Ambulatory blood pressure monitoring and postprandial hypotension in elderly patients with isolated systolic hypertension. *J Hum Hypertens* 1998; **12**:161–5.

Groppelli A, Giorgi DMA, Omboni S, Parati G, Mancia G. Persistant blood pressure increase induced by heavy smoking. *J Hypertens* 1992; **10**:495–9.

Grossman E, Messerli FH. Effect of calcium antagonists on plasma norepinephrine levels, heart rate, and blood pressure. *Am J Cardiol* 1997; **80**:1453–8.

Hakim AA, Petrovitch H, Burchfiel CM, et al. Effects of walking on mortality among nonsmoking retired men. *N Engl J Med* 1998; **338**:94–9.

Hall CL, Higgs CMB, Notarianni L. Home blood pressure recording in mild hypertension: value of distinguishing sustained from clinic hypertension and effect on diagnosis and treatment. *J Hum Hypertens* 1990; **4**:501–7.

Hallock P. Benson IC. Studies of the elastic properties of human isolated aorta. *J Clin Invest* 1937; **16**:595–602.

Hansson L, Zanchetti A, Carruthers SG  et al. Effects of intensive blood-pressure lowering and low-dose aspirin in patients with hypertension: principal results of the hypertension optimal treatment (HOT) randomised trial. *Lancet* 1998; **351**:1755–62.

Haynes RB, McKibbon KA, Kanani R. Systematic review of randomised trials of interventions to assist patients to follow prescriptions for medications. *Lancet* 1996; **348**:383–6.

Heikinheimo RJ, Haavisto MV, Kaarela RH et al. Blood pressure in the very old. *J Hypertens* 1990; **8**:361–7.

Huang Z, Willett WC, Manson JE. Body weight, weight change and risk for hypertension in women. *Ann Intern Med* 1998; 128:81–8.

Jackson R, Barham P, Biels J et al. Management of raised blood pressure in New Zealand: a discussion document. *BMJ* 1993; **307**:107–10.

Johnson AG. NSAIDS and blood pressure. *Drugs & Aging* 1998; **12**:17–27.

Joint National Committee. The sixth report of the Joint National Committee on detection, evaluation, and treatment of high blood pressure (JNC-VI). *Arch Intern Med* 1997; **157**:2413–46.

Jones JK, Gorkin L, Lian JF et al. Discontinuation of and changes in treatment after start of new courses of antihypertensive drugs: a study of a United Kingdom population. *BMJ* 1995; **311**:293–95.

Kannel WB. Prospects for prevention of cardiovascular disease in the elderly. *Prev Cardiol.* 1998; **1**:32-39.

Kaplan NM. Primary Hypertension: Pathogenesis. In: Kaplan NM, ed. *Clinical Hypertension*, 7th Edn. Baltimore: Williams & Wilkins 1998. 41–99.

Keith NM, Wagener HP, Barker NW. Some different types of essential hypertension: thier course and prognosis. *Am J Med Sci* 1937; **197**: 332–43

Langer RD, Criqui MH, Barrett-Connor EL et al. Blood pressure change and survival after age 75. *Hypertens* 1993; **22**:551–9.

Lieber MM. Pharmacologic therapy for prostatism. *Mayo Clin Proc* 1998; **73**:590–6

Lipsitz LA, Stouch HA, Manikear KL, Rowe JW Intra-individual varibility in postural BP in the elderly. *Clin Sci* 1985; **69**: 337–41

MacMahon S, Peto R, Cutler J et al. Blood pressure, stroke, and coronary heart disease. Part 1, Prolonged differences in blood pressure: prospective observational studes corrected for the regression dilution bias. *Lancet* 1990; **335**:765–74.

Mancia G, Sega R, Milesi C et al. Blood pressure control in the hypertensive population. *Lancet* 1997; **349**:454–7.

MRC Working Party. Medical Research Council trial of treatment of hypertension in older patients. *BMJ* 1992; **304**: 405–12.

Messerli FH, Grossman E, Goldbourt U. Are β-blockers efficacious as first-line therapy for hypertension in the elderly? *JAMA* 1998; **279**:1903–7.

Monane M, Bohn RL, Gurwitz JH et al. The effects of initial drug choice and comorbidity on antihypertensive therapy compliance. *Am J Hypertens* 1997; **10**:697–704.

Mulrow CD, Cornell JA, Herrera CR et al. Hypertension in the elderly. *JAMA* 1994; **272**:1932–38.

Neaton JD, Wentworth D. Serum cholesterol blood pressure, cigarette smoking and death from coronary heart disease. Overall findings and differences by age for 316,099 white men. *Arch Intern Med* 1992; **152**:56–64.

O'Brien E. Ave atque vale: the centenary of clinical sphygmomanometry. *Lancet* 1996; **348**:1569–70.

Ofili EO, Cohen JD, St. Vrain JA, et al. Effect of treatment of isolated systolic hypertension on left ventricular mass. *JAMA* 1998; **279**:778–80

O'Rourke M. Mechanical principles in arterial disease. *Hypertension* 1995; **26**:2-9.

Pickering TG. Blood pressure monitoring outside the office for the evaluation of patients with resistant hypertension. *Hypertension* 1988; **11**:(suppl II):II96–II100.

Psaty BM, Smith NL, Siscovick DS et al. Health outcomes associated with antihypertensive therapies used as first-line agents. *JAMA* 1997; **277**:739–45.

Rochon PA, Gurwitz JH. Optimising drug treatment for elderly people: the prescribing cascade. *BMJ* 1997; **315**:1096–99.

Rosenberg L, Rao S, Palmer JR, et al. Calcium channel blockers and the risk of cancer. *JAMA* 1998; **279**:1000–4.

Sacks FM, Willett WC, Smith A et al. Effect on blood pressure of potassium, calcium and magnesium in women with low habitual intake. *Hypertension* 1998; **31**:131–38.

Savage PJ, Pressel SL, Curb JD, et al. Influence of long-term, low-dose, diuretic-based, antihypertension therapy on glucose, lipid, uric acid, and potassium levels in older men and women with isolated systolic hypertension. *Arch Intern Med* 1998; **158**: 741–51.

Schwartz SM, Ross R. Cellular poroliferation in atherosclerosis and hypertension. *Prog Cardiovasc Dis* 1985; **26**:355

Shaper Ag, Wannamethee G, Whincup P. Alcohol and blood pressure in middle aged British men. *J Hum Hypertens* 1988; **2**:71–8

SHEP Cooperative Research Group. Prevention of stroke by antihypertensive drug treatment in older persons with isolated systolic hypertension. *JAMA* 1991; **265**:3254–64

Staessen JA, Fagard R, Thijs L et al. Randomised double-blind comparison of placebo and active treatment of older patients with isolated systolic hypertension. *Lancet* 1997; **350**:757–64.

Stewart IMG. Relation of reduction in pressure to first myocardial infarction in patients receiving treatment for severe hypertension. *Lancet* 1979;**1**: 1861–5

Thun MJ, Peto R, Lopez AD et al. Alcohol consumption and mortality among middle-aged and elderly U.S. adults. *N Engl J Med* 1997; **337**:1705–14

Tonkin AL. Postural hypotension. *Med J Aust* 1995; **162**:436–38.

Verdecchia P, Schillaci G, Boldrini F et al. White coat hypertension. *Lancet* 1996; **348**:1443–5.

Weinberger MH, Fineberg NS. Sodium and volume sensitivity of blood pressure. Age and pressure change over time. *Hypertension* 1991; **18**:67–71.

Whelton PK, Appel LJ, Espeland MA, et al. Sodium reduction and weight loss in the treatment of hypertension in older persons. *JAMA* 1998; **279**:839–46.

Zachariah PK, Sheps SG, Smith RL. Defining the roles of home and ambulatory monitoring. *Diagnosis* 1988;**10**: 39–50

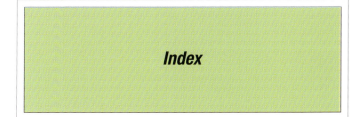

# *Index*

ACE inhibitors, see
    Angiotensin-converting
        enzyme inhibitors
Adherence, 90–3
Age
    antihypertensive
        therapy and, 61
        age limit, 62–3
    cardiovascular
        disease by, 21
    of onset, 16–17
    prevalence of hyper-
        tension by, 1
    systolic and diastolic
        BP by, 10
Alcohol intake, 74–5
Aldosteronism, primary,
    46
ALLHAT study, 58
Alpha-blockers, 85
Ambulatory/24 h (incl.-
    home) BP measure-
    ment, 23, 26, 87
    white coat effect and,
        27–30
Amiloride plus hydrochl-
    orothiazide, 56
Aneurysms
    aortic abdominal, 41,
        45
    retinal, 42, 43
Angiotensin II-receptor

blockers, 85–6
    renin levels and
        response to, 8
Angiotensin-converting
    enzyme inhibitors,
    85–6
    renin levels and
        response to, 7, 8
Antihypertensive and
    Lipid Lowering Heart
    Attack Prevention
    Trial, 58
Antihypertensive drugs,
    48–67, 78–89
    adverse effects, 78,
        79, 87–9
    on comorbid condi-
        tions, 83
    beneficial effects,
        48–67
    on comorbid condi-
        tions, 82, 85
    BP measurement
        and resistance to, 29
    compliance, 90–3
    goal, 64–7, 86
    guidelines, 80–9
        general, 80–6
        special, 86–9
    indications, 60–1, 80,
        82
    specific, 85–6

interactions, 87, 89
    renin levels and
        response to, 7–8
    trials, see Trials
    vascular dementia
        and, 22
    withdrawal in postural
        hypotension, 34
Aortic abdominal
    aneurysms, 41, 45
Aortic coarctation, 46
Apnea, sleep, 38
Apolipoprotein (a) levels,
    41
Arteries, large, changes
    in, 10–13
Arteriosclerosis, small
    vessel, 10
    retinopathy in, 40
Aspirin, 77
Assessment, patient,
    37–47
Atenolol trials, 53, 56, 80
    second-line, 54
Atherosclerosis, 10, 12
    renovascular disease
        in, 45

Baroreceptor activity,
    diminished, 78, 79
Bendrofluazide trial, 53
Beta-blockers, 59

renin levels and response to, 7, 8
special guidelines, 87
toxicity, 89
in trials, 59
first-line, 50, 53, 55–7, 59, 80
second-line, 54
Biochemical tests, *see* Laboratory tests
Black patients, renal damage, 6
Blood pressure diastolic, *see* Diastolic BP
measurement, 23–32
ambulatory/home, *see* Ambulatory BP measurement
errors, 32
systolic, *see* Systolic BP
Blood tests, *see* Laboratory tests

Calcium, dietary, 75
Calcium antagonists (long-acting dihydropyridines), 84–5
Chinese studies, 59, 84
HOT study, 65
renin levels and response to, 7, 8
special guidelines, 87
SYST-EUR study, *see* SYST-EUR
Cardiovascular events, risk of, 2, 18–21, 63, *see* also Heart attack of events
drug trials reducing, 48, 49, 50, 60
J-curve relating BP to, 64–6
in newly diagnosed hypertensives, 17, 18
in white coat and ambulatory hyperten-

sion, 29–30
Carotid bruit, 41
Cerebral autoregulation, impaired, 78, 79
Cerebral ischemia, symptoms, 41
Cerebrovascular disease (incl. stroke), risk of, 2, 18–19
drug trials reducing, 48, 49, 50, 60
Chinese trials
nifedipine, 59
nitrendipine, 59
Chlorthalidone trial, 54, 80
Cholesterol
raised levels, 40–1
reducing intake, 76
Clinical trials, *see* Trials
Compliance, 90–3
Conn syndrome (primary aldosteronism), 46
Coronary heart disease, *see* also Heart attack
death rates by systolic vs diastolic BP, 20 risk of 2,18–19, 20, 21
alcohol reducing (small amounts), 75
drug trials reducing, 48, 49, 50, 60
Cotton wool spots, 40, 43
Cuff size (BP measurement), 24
Cushing's syndrome, 46

Death/mortality rates
drug trials reducing, 60
in isolated systolic BP, 21
by systolic and diastolic BP, coronary heart disease and, 20, 21
in very elderly, 22
Definition, hypertension,

36
Dementia, vascular, 22
Diabetic hypertension, 85–6
HOT trial, 66
Diastolic BP
age and race and, 10
in definition of hypertension, 36
high, risk compared to systolic hypertension, 20
Diet
in history-taking, 38
modification, 70–6, 76–7
in postprandial hypotension, 36
sodium in, *see* Sodium
Dihydropyridines, *see* Calcium antagonists
Diuretics, 80–3
renin levels and response to, 7–8
special guidelines, 86–7
specific indications, 86
toxicity, 89
in trials, first-line, 48–9, 52-7, 60, 80–2
Drug therapy
in hypertension antihypertensives, *see* Antihypertensive drugs
other drugs, 77
in hypertension causation, 38
in postural hypotension, 34
Dyslipidemia, tests, 40–1

Eating, hypotension after, 33–6
ECG for left ventricular hypertrophy, 41, 44
Electrocardiography for

left ventricular hyper-
trophy, 41, 44
Enalapril, 57
Endothelial dysfunction,
5, 13–14
Epidemiology (incid-
ence/prevalence etc.)
hypertension, 1–2
postural and post-
prandial hypotension,
33
Equipment, BP mea-
surement, 24
Erectile failure, 88
Ethnicity, *see* Race
Etiology, *see*
Mechanisms
European Working Party
on Hypertension in
the Elderly trial, 52
Evaluation, patient,
37–47
EWPHE trial, 52
Examination, physical,
39–40
Exercise, 76

Family history, 38
Fat, saturated, reducing
intake, 76
Felodipine, HOT study,
65
Females, *see* Women
Food
hypotension after
eating, 33-6
sodium content, 72
Framingham data, 21
Funduscopy, 40, 42, 43

Gender, *see* Men;
Women
Genetic factors, 5

Heart
failure, congestive,
risk of, 2
ischemic disease, *see*
Coronary heart
disease

protective effect of
long-acting dihy-
dropyridines, 84
Heart attack, risk, 18
History, patient, 38–9
Home BP measurement,
*see* Ambulatory BP
measurement
Hormone replacement
therapy, 77
HOT trial, 65–7
HPE trial, 53
Hydrochlorothiazide (in
trial), 52
amiloride plus, 56
nitrendipine plus, 57
Hypercholesterolemia,
40–1
Hyperlipidemia, 41
Hypertension
definition, 36
"inappropriate", 44–5,
47
Hypertension Elderly
Patients trial, 53
Hypertension Optimal
Treatment, 65–7
Hypertriglyceridemia,
40-1
Hyperuricemia, 41
Hypotension
postprandial, 33-6
postural, 33–6, 67, 86

Impotence, 88
"Inappropriate" hyper-
tension, 44–5, 47
Incidence, *see*
Epidemiology
Ischemia, cerebral,
symptoms, 41
Ischemic heart disease,
*see* Coronary heart
disease

J-curve, 64–6
Joint National Comm-
ittee report (JNC-6)
on beta-blocker-based
trials, 59

on long-acting dihy-
dropyridines, 85
risk groups in, 61
treatment algorithm,
80, 81
Juxtaglomerular cells, 5,
7

Kidney, *see entries
under* Renal

Laboratory (incl. bio-
chemical) tests, 40–1
in SHEP trial, 80, 83
Large artery
changes, 10–13
Left ventricular hypert-
rophy, detection, 41
Lifestyle modification,
31, 68–77
Lipid abnormalities,
tests, 40–1
Lipoprotein (a) levels, 41
Loop diuretics in renal
insufficiency, 86

Magnesium, dietary, 75
Males, *see* Men
Management, *see*
Therapy
Manometer, 24
Mechanisms (etiology
and pathogenesis)
hypertension, 4–15
search for unusual
causes, 44–6
postural and post
prandial hypotension,
34–6
Medical Research
Council trial, 56, 80
Men, age and/or race in
cardiovascular dis-
ease by, 21
prevalence of hyper-
tension by, 1
systolic/diastolic BP
by, 10
MRC trial, 56, 80
MRFIT, 20

Multiple Risk Factor
    Intervention trial, 20
Myocardial infarction
    (heart attack), risk, 18

Natural history
    untreated hyper-
        tension, 17
    white-coat hyper-
        tension, 20–1
Nephron number,
    reduced, 5
Nephrosclerosis, benign,
    5–6
Nifedipine, Chinese
    study, 59
Nitrendipine
    Chinese study, 59
    European study, see
        SYST-EUR
Nitric oxide, 13, 14
Non-compliance, 90–3
Non-steroidal anti-
    inflammatory drugs
    and antihyper-
    tensives, 87, 88

Obesity/overweight, 5
    losing weight, 70
Oestrogen replacement
    therapy, 77
Ophthalmoscopy (fun-
    duscopy), 40, 42, 43
Optic disc abnormalities,
    40, 42, 43
Organ damage, target,
    63
    detecting, 41
    symptoms, 38
Orthostatic (postural)
    hypotension, 33–6,
    67, 86
Overweight, see Obesity

Pathogenesis, see
    Mechanisms
Pheochromocytoma, 46
Physical examination,
    39–40
Physical exercise, 76

Postprandial hypo-
    tension, 33–6
Postural hypotension,
    33–6, 67, 86
Posture and BP mea-
    surement, 24
Potassium, dietary, 75
Prevalence, see
    Epidemiology
Prostatism and alpha-
    blockers, 85
Pseudohypertension, 32
Psychosocial factors, 38
Pulse wave velocity, 13,
    14

Race/ethnicity
    prevalence of hyper-
        tension by, 1
    renal damage and, 6
    systolic and diastolic
        BP by, 10
Randomized controlled
    trials, see Trials
Renal development in
    small-for-gestational
    age babies, 6
Renal disease
    (damage/dysfunction),
    hypertensive, 5–6
    detection, 41, 46
Renal insufficiency, loop
    diuretics, 86
Renin, 5–8
Renovascular disease,
    atherosclerotic, 45
Reserpine, 54
Resistant hypertension,
    BP measurement
    and, 29
Retinopathy, 40, 42, 43
Risk (of complications),
    2, 16-22, see also
        specific risks
    reduction in drug
        trials, 48, 49, 50, 60
    risk stratification and
        drug therapy, 61,
        62
    white coat hyper-

tension and, 32
Risk factors for hyper-
    tension, 63
    in history-taking, 38

Salt, dietary, see
    Sodium, dietary
Saturated fat intake,
    reducing, 76
Sex, see Men; Women
Shanghai Trial of
    Nifedipine in the
    Elderly, 59
SHEP, see Systolic
    Hypertension in the
    Elderly Program
Sildenafil, 88
Sleep apnea, 38
Small-for-gestational age
    babies, renal develop-
    ment, 6
Small vessel arteriosc-
    lerosis, see Arterio-
    sclerosis
Smoking, stopping, 69
Sodium, dietary
    intake
        excess, 5
        restriction, 70–4
    sensitivity to,
        increased, 8–9, 71
Sphygmomanometer, 24
    artefactual readings,
    32
Stethoscope, 25
STONE trial, 59
STOP-HT, 55
Stress, 5
Stroke, see
    Cerebrovascular
    disease
Swedish Trial in Old
    Patients with
    Hypertension, 55
Symptoms in history-
    taking, 38
Syst-China trial, 59
SYST-EUR (nitrendipine)
    trial, 50, 57, 58, 85
    vascular dementia

and, 22
Systolic BP
    age and race and, 10
    high (systolic hyper-
        tension), 9-13
        definition, 36
        isolated, mortality
            rates, 21
        risk compared to
            diastolic hyper-
            tension, 20
Systolic Hypertension in
    Europeans study, *see*
    SYST-EUR
Systolic Hypertension in
    the Elderly Program
    (SHEP), 54, 67,
    80-2
    postural hypotension,
        33

Therapy
    hypertension, 3,
    48-93
        benefits, 48-67
        drug therapy, *see*
            Antihypertensive
            drugs
        non-drug therapy,
            31, 68-77
    hypotension
        postprandial, 36
        postural, 34
Thiazide diuretics, 80-3,
    86
    toxicity, 89
    trials, 52-7
Tobacco avoidance, 69
TONE trial, 72-4
Treatment, *see* Therapy
Trials, randomized con-
    trolled, *see also spe-
    cific trials*
    dietary modification,
        72-4
    drugs, 48-67, 80-2,
        84-5
Triamterene trial, 52
Triglycerides, raised,
    40-1

Uric acid, raised, 41

Vascular dementia, 22
Vascular endothelial
    dysfunction, 5, 13-14
Ventricular hypertrophy,
    left, detection, 41
Very elderly, 22
Viagra, 88

Weight loss, 70
White coat effects/hyper-
    tension, 27-32
Women
    age and/or race in
        cardiovascular
        disease by, 21
    prevalence of
        hypertension by, 1
        systolic/diastolic
        BP by, 10
    oestrogen replace-
        ment therapy, 77